CW00428713

The
Midwifery R___
Database
MIRIAD

MIC INFORMATION SERV
Allerton P

Third Edition

*A sourcebook of information about
research in midwifery*

'5

Edited by
Felicia McCormick
Mary J. Renfrew

Books for Midwives Press
nd Limited

05626420

Published by Books for Midwives Press, 174a Ashley Road, Hale, Cheshire, WA15 9SF, England.

© 1997, Crown copyright. Published by permission of the Northern and Yorkshire Regional Office, National Health Service Executive. No part of this publication may be reproduced in any form without the permission of the Northern and Yorkshire Regional Office, National Health Service Executive.

First edition.

All rights reserved. No part of this book may be reproduced in any form or by any electronic or mechanical means, including information storage and retrieval systems, without permission in writing from the publisher, except by a reviewer who may quote passages in a review.

ISBN 1-898507-63-5

British Library Cataloguing in Publication Data
A catalogue record for this book is available from the British Library

Printed in Great Britain by Redwood Books, Trowbridge, Wiltshire.

A•I•S	
STOCK No.	
SITE	AL
CLASS No.	618.20072
SUFFIX	MID

National Research Register

The National Research Register (NRR) is a user friendly database containing information about Research and Development (R & D) projects which are currently taking place in or are of interest to the NHS.

To get details of your project onto the NRR you should make contact with the Information Manager of R & D at your NHS Executive Regional Office.

Contents

Acknowledgements

Many people have given their time and expertise to the preparation of this report. Especially important have been the researchers who have provided details about their studies, and who responded to our many requests for additional information.

Julie Batchelor has played an essential role in the project and is much missed having left for a full time post. Many thanks!

We welcome Jenny Padgham, who joined us in January 1997 and has helped with the final stages of preparing this report.

We are grateful for the continuing help and support of our Advisory Group.

Our thanks again to Henry Hochland, Catherine Bryant, Emma Gallaway and colleagues at Hochland and Hochland Ltd.

We thank Mike Kelly, our software consultant, and all our colleagues at Midwifery Studies and at the Division of Midwifery, who give us great support.

Since the last report the project has moved offices and we are grateful to the University of Leeds for our comfortable new accommodation.

By funding the database since May 1996, Northern and Yorkshire Region has enabled The Midwifery Research Database, MIRIAD to continue its work for a further eighteen months. We are enormously grateful for this.

The publication of this report has been made possible by an additional grant from the Department of Health.

Staff and Advisory Group Members 1995–1997

Staff

Julie Batchelor	Secretary (until October 1996)
Felicia McCormick	Database Administrator
Jenny Padgham	Database Coordinator (from January 1997)
Mary Renfrew	Professor of Midwifery Studies

Advisory group members

Elisabeth Clark	Royal College of Nursing
Sue Hawkins	Midwives Information and Resource Service
Hazel McHaffie	University of Edinburgh
Kathryn Partington	Department of Health
Louise Silverton	Royal College of Midwives (until March 1997)
Jennifer Sleep	Thames Valley University
Rosaline Steele	Royal College of Midwives (from March 1997)
Ann Thomson	University of Manchester

National Research Register

The National Research Register (NRR) is a user friendly database containing information about Research and Development (R & D) projects which are currently taking place in or are of interest to the NHS.

To get details of your project onto the NRR you should make contact with the Information Manager of R & D at your NHS Executive Regional Office.

Introduction

Mothers and babies should receive the best possible maternity care. To provide that care, midwives and other caregivers, managers and policy makers, as well as childbearing women, need up to date evidence about the effects of care. Excellent sources of such information exist and some of them are listed on p.ix of this Introduction. However the need and demand for good quality, up to date, comprehensive and easily accessible information about the effects of care is growing and will continue to grow.

Since 1988 The Midwifery Research Database, MIRIAD has provided information about both published and unpublished, completed and ongoing research in the field of midwifery, and has set up a network of researchers willing to respond to queries about their research.

This is the fifth report of the information held on the database, and the third to be published by Books for Midwives Press. As a result of our arrangement with Books for Midwives Press, the book has become much more widely available. This report has been produced with the help of additional funding from the Department of Health. MIRIAD must now find ways of providing information about research in midwifery to our users which meet their needs, whilst being less costly both to collate and to disseminate.

In February 1997 we conducted a user survey to guide us as to how we can best contribute to meeting our reader's requirements. As a result of this, we are now planning to produce data from MIRIAD in a condensed form, as a register. The price of this report includes a six month subscription to the register. Your feedback about the form and content of the register will be invaluable for its successful development. To claim your free subscription complete the card inserted at the back of this book.

The development of MIRIAD

The Midwifery Research Database, MIRIAD, is a unique compilation of information about ongoing and completed research in midwifery. Since 1988, details about midwifery research studies in the UK have been collected on a computerised database run until 1994 by the Midwifery Research Programme at the National Perinatal Epidemiology Unit in Oxford and since 1995 from Midwifery Studies at the University of Leeds where Mary Renfrew was appointed as Chair in 1994. Details of studies in clinical practice, midwifery education, the organisation of midwifery services and the history of midwifery are all included. This is the only source of information about much of this work – almost a fifth of the studies (68, 19%) are still in progress, and many of the completed studies have never been published elsewhere.

MIRIAD is now funded by Northern and Yorkshire Region.

Finding MIRIAD studies

When this book went to press there were 374 midwifery research studies registered with MIRIAD. To find those studies, we generated publicity about the database each year in professional and research journals, and at relevant conferences. Researchers were asked to contact us for a registration form. They then returned that form to the MIRIAD office, giving details about their study. If the criteria for entry to the database were fulfilled (see below) their studies were entered on to the computer, and examined for accuracy and completeness. A printout was then sent back to the researchers for checking.

Criteria for entry to MIRIAD

1. All studies are or were carried out in the United Kingdom.

2. Each study is related to midwifery but the researchers may or may not be midwives.

3. Quality assurance/audit projects are not included.
    Although quality assurance and research are sometimes closely related, the decision was made not to include quality assurance projects unless they involved directly some element of research.

4. Studies are not generally included if they were done as part of a student project at lower than undergraduate level.
    This is to exclude projects whose primary purpose was as a learning experience for the student, rather than as a research study. However, in exceptional cases, this criterion has been waived.

This edition includes updates for 22 of the 61 studies ongoing in the Second Edition (1996) and 29 new studies, whose entries were finalized by 10 October 1996. Studies whose completed abstract has appeared in a previous edition do not appear here. Readers who wish to have a complete record of all the studies will need a copy of MIRIAD 1994 and all our subsequent reports.

The studies vary widely in scale, method and quality. They have not undergone peer review unless they have already been published in refereed journals. Further investigation by the reader will be needed, including critical reading of any publications, or contacting the researchers involved, to assess the quality of the study. In addition, the studies reported here may not be the only relevant work - there may be important studies which are not listed here, and there may be studies in fields other than midwifery which are also important. All relevant work on a particular topic should be explored before implementing changes in practice. Ways of finding information about other work are outlined below.

Further information about published studies in midwifery can be obtained from:

> *Midwives Information and Resource Service (MIDIRS), 9 Elmdale Road, Clifton, Bristol, BS8 1SL. Tel: **0800 581009 (freephone)** email: **midirs@dial.pipex.com** internet address: **http://www.gn.apc.org/midirs***

and from:

> *Royal College of Midwives Library, 15 Mansfield Street, London W1M 0BE. Tel: **(0171) 872 5160**.*

*Other important sources of information include libraries, computerized indexes such as MEDLINE, and the computerized database of reviews of perinatal trials, 'The Cochrane Collaboration Pregnancy and Childbirth Module', edited by Murray Enkin, Marc Keirse, Mary Renfrew and James Neilson, issued on disk twice yearly as part of 'The Cochrane Library' by BMJ Publishing Group, PO Box 295, London WC1H 9TE. Tel: **(0171) 383 6185/6245** Fax: **(0171) 383 6662**.*

Further information about clinical audit in maternity services can be obtained from:

> *Angie Benbow and Julie Wray, Audit Unit, St. Mary's Hospital, Hathersage Road, Manchester M13 0JH. Tel: **(0161) 276 6300** Fax: **(0161) 276 6311**.*

Since this manuscript went to press, further studies have been submitted to us. It is important that we collect information about as many studies as possible, so that this book is really useful to the readers. Information about completed or ongoing studies in midwifery will always be welcome.

We rely completely on researchers sending us details of their research; if they do not, we cannot enter their study on to the database.

If you have a study which you would like to register, please contact us at:

MIRIAD,
Midwifery Studies, University of Leeds,
22 Hyde Terrace, Leeds, LS2 9LN.
Tel: (0113) 233 6886 Fax: (0113) 244 9730
email: f.m.mccormick@leeds.ac.uk

and ask for Felicia McCormick or Jenny Padgham.

Summary of information about midwifery research studies

Completed and ongoing studies

This is the Third Edition (1997) of The Midwifery Research Database, MIRIAD. Of the 51 studies listed here 29 are new, and 22 have had their entries updated since they appeared in the Second Edition (1996). Thirty two studies have been completed and are listed in full. Twenty one of these have been newly entered with MIRIAD as completed studies and 11 studies have been completed since the Second Edition. Nineteen studies (8 new and 11 updated) are ongoing. Studies whose entries were complete in MIRIAD 1994 or in the Second Edition (1996) are not reported here. Interested readers should refer to the earlier publications for details of these studies. All contact details for researchers have been updated and the MIRIAD office can forward enquiries about previously completed studies to researchers.

For simplicity, the following tables and text will refer to the three MIRIAD reports published by Books for Midwives Press as follows: MIRIAD 1994 (the First Edition), MIRIAD 1996 (the Second Edition) and MIRIAD 1997 (this book, the Third Edition).

Categories of study

There are four main categories of study: Clinical, Educational, Management and Historical. MIRIAD staff allocate these categories according to the subject area(s) covered by each study. A study may fall into more than one category; for example, it may be about the effect of education on clinical practice. If this is the case, it will be listed in full in the most appropriate section, and cross-referenced to other relevant sections.

Table 1: Numbers of studies in each category in MIRIAD 1996 and 1997

Category	1996 n=345[1]		1997 n=29[2]	
	No.	%	No.	%
Clinical	270	78	23	79
Educational	62	18	4	14
Management	85	25	2	7
Historical	4	1	0	0
Totals [3]	421		29	

[1]   MIRIAD 1996 included all studies reported in MIRIAD 1994, except for 22 listed as 'Studies which will not be completed' (MIRIAD 1996 p.371).

[2]   These studies were entered and had their entries finalized between 18 August 1995 and 10 October 1996.

[3]   Note that some studies appear in more than one category.

Table 1 shows the numbers of studies in each category in MIRIAD 1996 and 1997. None of the studies in MIRIAD 1997 fall into the Historical category. There has been an increase in the numbers of studies in the other categories, with no disproportionate increase in any one category. The great majority of studies falling into more than one category combine clinical and management topics.

Keywords

Each study has been allocated a maximum of 10 keywords by the researchers or by MIRIAD staff. These have been used to compile the index, and to indicate the frequency with which topics occur.

Excluding the term 'midwifery', which is of course used in a very large number of studies, the keywords which were used most frequently are as shown in Table 2.

Table 2: Most frequently used keywords in MIRIAD 1996 and 1997

Keywords used[1]	Number of Entries	
	1996 n=345	*1997 n=29*
Labour	116	5
Breastfeeding	113	16
Midwifery education	108	14
Women's experience	55	9
Antenatal care	52	1
Perineal care	49	1
Postnatal care	39	1
Consumer satisfaction	38	1
Midwives' role	32	1
Maternity services	28	1
Student midwives	21	3
Continuity of care	20	1

[1] including closely related keywords

Breastfeeding, labour, antenatal care and perineal care were the most frequently mentioned clinical topics in all the previous MIRIAD reports and this remains the same in this edition. The order of the top three keywords used has returned to that of the MIRIAD 1994. Studies concerned with midwifery education and women's experience have increased approximately in line with the increase in total studies sent to MIRIAD. The range of questions addressed in the 29 new studies is wide and many other keywords have been used once or twice only. Several new keywords have been added, including diet, and termination of pregnancy (both used twice).

Timing of studies

Table 3 shows when the studies were started.

Table 3: Starting date of studies reported in MIRIAD 1996 and 1997

Year	1996 (n=345)	1997 (n=29)
1975 and before	1	0
1976 to 1980	21	0
1981 to 1985	40	1
1986 to 1990	115	2
1991 to 1995	168 [1]	24
1996	N/A	4 [2]

[1] Entries finalized by 18 August 1995
[2] Entries finalized by 10 October 1996

Most studies included for the first time in MIRIAD 1996 and 1997 were current or recently completed.

Were studies carried out in work time?

Researchers were asked whether the person who carried out the study did so as part of a job, in her/his own time, or as part of a course. Table 4 gives the answers to this question. The responses are not mutually exclusive; for example, some researchers may have carried out a study which formed part of a course, as well as part of their job, and additionally have spent some of their own time working on it.

Table 4: Were studies carried out in work time?

	1996 (n=345)		1997 (n=29)	
	No.	%	No.	%
As integral or additional part of a job	209	60	14	48
Outside work time	136	39	20	69
As part of a course	149	43	14	48
Other/Don't know	29	8	1	3

It has not been possible accurately to differentiate between an integral and an additional part of a job, often because those carrying out the research themselves have difficulty deciding where the scope of their job ended. For example, some researchers used the clinical facilities in which they were working to carry out their study, but additionally used their own time outside their normal duties. Others carried out a study in their normal hours, but with an increased workload as a result. Full-time researchers, especially, had difficulty in differentiating between normal and additional parts of a job; the hours worked by researchers are not usually rigidly defined, and work is often done at home. Table 4 shows that a higher percentage of researchers reported using some time outside work on studies entered in MIRIAD 1997. However, only one of these 29 studies was neither part of a job nor part of a course. Researchers seem to be negotiating some work time or study leave for their research, even if it is not part of their current job. This suggests increased commitment on the part of midwifery managers to supporting research activity.

Table 5 shows the average amount of time principal researchers used outside their work hours throughout the study. This figure is hard for those involved in the research to estimate, for some of the reasons outlined above. In addition, research does not happen at a steady pace, and more time will be spent in some phases of a study than in others.

Table 5: Time spent by principal researchers outside their work hours

Average no. of hours/week	1996 (n=345)		1997 (n=29)	
	No.	%	No.	%
Less than 2 hours	25	7	4	14
2 to 6 hours	67	19	8	28
7 to 12 hours	63	18	3	10
13 to 20 hours	33	9	2	7
More than 20 hours	22	6	3	10
None of their own time/don't know	135	39	9	31
Total who used their own time	210	59	20	69

These results indicate that being involved in research eats substantially into the majority of researchers' own time, with 15 per cent up to August 1995 and 17 per cent of those registering later spending more than an additional 12 hours a week on their studies.

Sources of funding

Questions about the way the study was funded are also difficult to answer. Does 'funding' include material support, such as stationery and photocopying, or time release from work? Researchers seemed to answer this question in a variety of ways, and as a result it is not possible to make any definitive statement about how studies were funded. Table 6 gives such information as is available about sources of funding: some studies had more than one source of funding, and some funding agencies are also employers, so the answers are not mutually exclusive. These figures probably underestimate funding support, as they do not always include estimates of integral costs such as time allowed at work. In addition, many of the researchers who reported receiving support also funded parts of their own studies, in time or money. Those coded 'other source' were simply impossible to categorize in any straightforward way. Some of these researchers requested that we keep the source of funding confidential. Others found it hard to work out, for example, how much of an award for educational support was spent on their study.

Table 6: Source of funding for studies

Source of funding for studies	1996 n=345		1997 n=29	
	No.	%	No.	%
Employer	175	51	20	69
Funding agency	136	39	15	52
Other source	46	13	1	3
No funding received	51	15	5	17
No response	2	0.6	0	0

Table 6 shows that MIRIAD 1997 includes a greater percentage of studies funded by a funding agency than have our previous reports. This follows more than sixty requests for registration forms for new studies from researchers who already had a study registered with MIRIAD, when they updated their contact details after the publication of MIRIAD 1996. This may be an indication of developing maturity in research in midwifery.

Finding funds for research remains difficult, perhaps especially so in midwifery where there are few obvious sources of appropriate support. Organizations which did contribute funds to studies included for the first time in MIRIAD 1997 are indexed on p.126–27.

Ethics committee approval

Eighteen of the 29 new studies in MIRIAD 1997 (62 per cent) reported that they had gained ethics committee approval, and 11 (38 per cent) had not. In MIRIAD 1994 and in MIRIAD 1996 these percentages were 60 per cent and 40 per cent respectively. Many of these researchers asked permission from other sources, such as the Director of Midwifery Services, instead of applying to an Ethics Committee. Others felt that ethics approval was not needed for their study. In some studies this was because those being interviewed were health professionals rather than women themselves. One study is a systematic review and another is a secondary analysis of data. In other circumstances, it was not clear why the researcher felt that ethics committee approval was not required. For example, some researchers collected information from case notes, and others interviewed women individually and in groups, without having requested ethics committee approval.

Study design

Information was requested about the study design. One question asked whether the study was descriptive or experimental. Researchers for three of the new studies in MIRIAD 1997 (10 per cent) noted that their study was experimental (27 per cent in 1994, 19 per cent in MIRIAD 1996) and 24 (83 per cent) carried out a descriptive study (79 per cent in 1994, 75 per cent in MIRIAD 1996).

Research method

The study abstracts published in MIRIAD 1994 were presented in one of two formats. One hundred and thirty nine appeared in the free text format of earlier MIRIAD publications, and 128 as structured abstracts - the format now used for all MIRIAD study entries. Researchers who completed a structured abstract were asked for details about research methods used in their studies. Table 7 gives details about the research method used in studies with structured abstracts. More than one method might be used within a single study; some studies consist of several interconnected parts involving different methods. Examples of methods used in the 'other' category include experimental studies (other than randomized controlled trials), systematic reviews, case note reviews, analysis of documents, critical literature review, Grounded Theory, critical incident technique and group discussions.

Table 7: Research method used

Research method	Structured abstracts 1994 and 1996 (n=227)		Structured abstracts 1997 (n=29)	
	No.	%	No.	%
Survey	118	52	17	59
Ethnography/ phenomenology	32	14	3	10
Case Study	22	10	2	7
Historical study	7	3	0	0
Randomized controlled trial	38	17	2	7
Case control	7	3	1	3
Action research	11	5	1	3
Other	47	21	6	21
No response	1	0.4	0	0

Finally, many of the completed studies have not been published. It is understandable that many researchers, working under pressure, with scarce resources, and without good supervision, find it hard to find the time to finish a study. A survey of these researchers has been carried out to ascertain some of the reasons for this lack of publication; the results are being analysed.

In conclusion

The work presented in this report demonstrates continued growth in research in midwifery, and in the variety of topics being addressed.

Some problems highlighted in MIRIAD 1996 remain. Some researchers have not sought ethics committee approval even when this seemed to be appropriate. Among the ongoing studies which have not been updated it appears that some will not be completed, possibly because of a lack of support and advice, or funding, or perhaps because inappropriate questions were asked. Other studies have been completed but not published; we plan to clarify the reasons for this.

These problems need to be addressed by the midwifery profession, by managers, researchers and funding bodies.

The questions being addressed in the research presented here are of importance to women, their babies and their families, as well as to midwives, and others working in the maternity services. We plan to demonstrate how this work has developed in future publications.

Listing of individual studies

Full details of all studies in MIRIAD are given under four main headings; Clinical, Educational, Management and Historical. Where study topics relate to more than one category the full record appears in the most appropriate category and is cross referenced to any other relevant category. Most of the entries are in the Clinical section, and for this edition these have been grouped in subject order. Entries in the Educational and Management sections are listed as in previous editions in order of their study number; this number was allocated chronologically, as studies were entered on the database. There were no studies in the Historical category for the Third Edition.

The study number and title are listed first, followed by the dates during which the study was/is being carried out. The researchers names and job titles are next. The first name listed is usually that of the person who had/has principal responsibility for the study. The person who is willing to be contacted about the study is listed as the Contact, followed by their address. This address is usually the person's current work address and is therefore not always the address of the institution where the study was carried out. Some researchers cannot be contacted at work, and therefore contact with them should be made via the MIRIAD Office. This is indicated on their entries. Our contact details are:

MIRIAD
Midwifery Studies
22 Hyde Terrace
Leeds LS2 9LN

Tel: (0113) 233 6886
Fax: (0113) 244 9730
E-mail f.m.mccormick@leeds.ac.uk

When writing to a researcher, whether directly or c/o the MIRIAD office, it is helpful to enclose a stamped addressed envelope for their reply.

Job titles have been updated where possible, and are therefore for current jobs, for the principal researcher (who is listed first), and the contact person. Collaborators' job titles are those which were current at the time of the study.

Funding details are then given. Key words are listed next; these correspond to those listed in the key word index, and will assist in identifying studies of interest. The study abstracts follow. Finally, any publications or reports from the study are cited in full.

At the back of the report there is an author index and a keyword index, both listed alphabetically, to help you find studies of interest.

Note: MIRIAD is not intended to provide a direct basis for changing practice. Studies entered on MIRIAD have not undergone peer review unless they have been published in refereed journals. Further investigation by the reader will be required in all instances, to assess the quality of the study. In addition, the studies reported here may not be the only relevant work in the field, and it is important to explore all the work on a particular topic before implementing change.

Title index

Clinical studies: before and during pregnancy

374. ADOLESCENTS' PERCEPTIONS OF HEALTHY PREGNANCY
March 1995–December 1995

Grace Edwards, Martin Stanisstreet, Edward Boyes. **Contact:** Grace Edwards, Perinatal Surveys Manager, Unit of Perinatal and Paediatric Epidemiology, Department of Public Health, Muspratt Building, University of Liverpool, Liverpool L69 3BX. Tel: (0151) 794 5276. Fax: (0151) 794 5270. Email: grace@liv.ac.uk.

Funded as integral/additional part of a job by funding agency: North West Regional Health Authority, Small Grants and Research Committee. 6–12 hours/week of own time spent.

Keywords: ADOLESCENTS, ANTENATAL EDUCATION, EDUCATION FOR PARENTHOOD, PREGNANCY

Aims of the study:
To determine the ideas of adolescents about how a woman's lifestyle during pregnancy can affect fetal well being.

Ethics committee approval gained:
No

Research design:
Descriptive, qualitative, quantitative, survey.

> **Data Collection:**
> > **Techniques used:**
> > > Semistructured interviews, open format qualitative questionnaires, and final closed format quantitative questionnaires.
>
> > **Time data were collected:**
> > > During the spring and summer school terms of 1995.
>
> > **Testing of any tools used:**
> > > Interviews piloted with 10 children, open questionnaires with 100 children and closed questionnaires with 93 children.
>
> > **Topics covered:**
> > > What women should eat, drink and do preconceptually.
> > > What pregnant women should eat, drink and do.
>
> > **Setting for data collection:**
> > > Urban and rural secondary schools.
>
> **Details about sample studied:**
> > **Planned size of sample:**
> > > No planned size for interviews
> > > >300 for open questionnaire and >600 for closed questionnaire.
>
> > **Rationale for planned size:**
> > > As large as possible.

Entry criteria:
Inclusion:

All children were in national curriculum year 10 at mixed gender, non-religious community comprehensive schools.

Exclusion:

Single sex, religious, private sector and selective schools.

Sample selection:

All available secondary schools in the area which met the criteria.

Actual sample size:

44 interviews, 404 open questionnaires and 708 closed questionnaires.

Interventions, Outcomes and Analysis:
Analysis:

Closed questionnaires analysed for consistency and reliability, interviews and open questionnaires coded and concepts analysed, all using SPSS.

Results:
Children were well informed on some aspects of healthy pregnancy, especially alcohol and smoking, but knew little of the risks to the fetus from specific items, e.g. salmonella from eggs, vitamin A excess from liver or listeria from unpasteurized dairy products. The majority of children thought that the time to start 'taking care' was as soon as pregnancy is confirmed, suggesting they have little knowledge of preconceptual or periconceptual health.

Recommendations from this study:
Even if young peoples' knowledge about diet and actions for a healthy pregnancy is good, health outcomes will be frustrated if women do not respond until after the period of embryo vulnerability. There is a role for midwives in preconceptual education, which should be initiated for secondary school pupils.

Plans to continue in this area
The contact researcher intends to extend this research, including newly pregnant women, as part of a PhD.

426. SYSTEMATIC REVIEW OF RESEARCH EVIDENCE OF EFFECTIVENESS OF CURRENT INTERVENTIONS AIMING TO PROMOTE HEALTHIER EATING IN WOMEN OF CHILDBEARING AGE, AND THOSE WHO ARE PREGNANT
August 1996–January 1997

Edwin van Teijlingen, Lecturer, University of Aberdeen; Brenda J. Wilson, Lecturer, University of Aberdeen; Paul D. Lawrence, Librarian, University of Aberdeen; Doris M. Campbell, Senior Lecturer, University of Aberdeen; Ann Ralph, Assistant to the Director,

Rowett Research Unit, Aberdeen; Timothy P. Gill, Director of Postgraduate Education, Rowett Research Unit, Aberdeen; W. Philip T. James, Director, Rowett Research Unit, Aberdeen; Wendy J. Graham, Director, Dugald Baird Centre, University of Aberdeen. **Contact:** Edwin van Teijlingen, Department of Public Health, Medical School, University of Aberdeen, Aberdeen AB25 2ZD. Tel: (01224) 681818 ext. 52491.

Research commissioned and funded by a grant from the Health Education Authority. 2-6 hours per week of lead researcher's own time spent.

Keywords: DIET, HEALTH BEHAVIOUR, HEALTH BELIEFS, HEALTH EDUCATION, HEALTH PROMOTION, NUTRITION, PREGNANCY

Aims of the study:
This systematic review aims to collect research evidence of effectiveness of current health promotion interventions in the field of healthy eating in women of childbearing age and those who are pregnant.

Ethics committee approval gained:
No; not primary research.

Research design:
Systematic review (secondary research).

Data collection:
Techniques used:
Using the Cochrane Collaboration's guidelines we search through electronic databases, bibliographies of key articles and the grey literature to collect the most complete possible set of research findings in this field. The relevant papers will then be peer reviewed on the basis of predefined criteria. In addition, detailed data concerning the context of the study and characteristics of the intervention will be assessed by two reviewers.

Time data were collected:
1985-1996, retrospectively.

Testing of any tools used:
Checklist/schedule devised with funding body.

Topics covered:
Nutrition, diet, pregnancy, childbearing age, health promotion (diet only).

Setting for data collection:
University library.

Details about sample studied:
Planned size of sample:
Total available papers on topic from 1980.

Rationale for planned size:
> Few randomized controlled trials before 1980.

Entry criteria:
Inclusions:
> Papers published in or after 1980, reporting randomized controlled trials with groups of well women who are pregnant or of childbearing age.

Exclusions:
> Papers not in English; health promotion interventions with women who have a specific illness, or women who are breastfeeding.

Sample selection:
> See Data collection: Techniques used.

Actual sample size:
> Not yet known.

Response rate:
> N/A

Interventions, outcomes and analysis:
Analysis:
> Appraisal of abstracts and full papers. Information summarized on data abstract form schedule, assessed by two reviewers.

Results:
> In preparation.

416. A STUDY EXPLORING MIDWIVES' EDUCATION IN, KNOWLEDGE OF AND ATTITUDES TO NUTRITION IN PREGNANCY

June 1984–June 1985

Claire Mulliner, ex Staff Midwife, Helen Spiby, Midwifery Research Sister, Robert Fraser, Senior Lecturer. **Contact:** Helen Spiby, Midwifery Research Sister, Obstetrics and Gynaecology Management, First Floor Nurses' Home, Northern General Hospital, Herries Road, Sheffield S5 7AU. Tel: (0114) 271 4608.

Funded as integral part of a job by Evian/Birthright Health Bursary.

Keywords: ANTENATAL CARE, MIDWIFERY EDUCATION, MIDWIFERY EDUCATION (CONTINUING), MIDWIVES' ATTITUDES, NUTRITION

Aims of the study:
To explore the issues surrounding the nutritional knowledge of midwives, their education and their feelings about offering dietary advice to women in their care.

Ethics committee approval gained:
No. Not required by ethics committee for a study of midwives.

Research design:
Descriptive, qualitative and quantitative, survey.

Data collection:
Techniques used:
Questionnaires and interviews.

Time data were collected:
1984–5

Testing of any tools used:
Questionnaires and interview schedules piloted with 11 midwives.

Topics covered:
See Aims of the study.

Setting for data collection:
Midwives' work base.

Details about sample studied:
Planned size of sample:
77

Rationale for planned size:
10 per cent of registered midwives in one English Health Region.

Entry criteria:
Inclusions:
Registered midwives working in one English Health Region who consented to participate.

Sample selection:
Random.

Actual sample size:
58

Response rate:
58/77=75 per cent

Interventions, outcomes and analysis:
Analysis:
Frequencies and content analysis.

Results:
Midwife teachers were responsible for 95 per cent of teaching about nutrition. 86 per cent of respondents had received no education in nutrition following qualification. 46 per cent of respondents achieved a poor score in nutrition knowledge. Considerable numbers of respondents felt unprepared to offer dietary advice to women from ethnic minority groups (36 per cent), vegetarians (66 per cent), and to women with pre-existing medical conditions (41 per cent).

Recommendations from this study:
- Midwives require more education in nutrition both before and after qualification as midwives.
- Timely guidance on issues arising from 'food scares', in advance of media publicity, is needed.

Closer clinical links with dietetic departments, and increased dietetic involvement in midwifery education should be set up to meet these needs.

Suggestions for further research:
Replication with a group of newly qualified midwives, to gain information related to current midwifery education.

Develop and test a dietary advice pack for midwives.

Mulliner, C. M., Spiby, H., Fraser, R. B. (1995) 'A study exploring midwives' education in, knowledge of and attitudes to nutrition in pregnancy'. *Midwifery* 11, 37–41.

356. PREGNANCY RISK FACTORS FOR LEARNING DISABILITY IN CHILDHOOD
April 1994–December 1995

David K. James, Professor of Fetomaternal Medicine, University of Nottingham; Mitchel E. Blair, Senior Lecturer/Community Physician Child Health; Florence M. Telfer, Research Midwife; Mark A. Wilcox, Senior Registrar, Obstetrics and Gynaecology; Clair Chilvers, Professor of Epidemiology, University of Nottingham; Nicki Keating, Statistician, University of Nottingham. **Contact:** Florence M. Telfer, via MIRIAD office.

Funded as integral/additional part of a job by Trent Regional Health Authority.

Keywords: ANTENATAL SCREENING, COMPUTERIZATION (OBSTETRIC RECORDS), HIGH RISK PREGNANCY, OUTCOMES (PAEDIATRIC), SPECIAL NEEDS, SPECIAL NEEDS REGISTER

Aims of the study:
That a cohort of women can be identified during pregnancy as being at greater risk of having a child with subsequent learning difficulties than the general Nottingham pregnant population.

Ethics committee approval gained:
No

Research design:
Descriptive, quantitative, case control study.

Data Collection:
Techniques used:
>Database records from the obstetric and Special Needs Registers (SNR). Case note review was reserved for cases not entered on the obstetric database.

Time data were collected:
>Retrospectively.

Testing of any tools used:
>Pilot study carried out to test the statistical methods.

Topics covered:
>Demographic data
>Anthropometric data
>Pregnancy and childbirth data

Setting for data collection:
>Hospital and community settings.

Details about sample studied:
Planned size of sample:
>540 study cases.

Rationale for planned size:
>Number of children born in Nottingham and entered on the SNR for the period 1987–93.

Entry criteria:
Inclusion:
>All children born in Nottingham and entered on the SNR 1987–93.

Exclusion:
>Multiple pregnancies excluded, but compiled as a subset of the main group.

Sample selection:
>Convenience.

Actual sample size:
>461 study cases. 461 control cases.

Response rate:
87 per cent.

Interventions, Outcomes and Analysis:
   Analysis:
   Two methods used:
   1.   Univariate analysis to identify any significant obstetric factor
   2.   Multivariate analysis to identify any significant independent risk.

   Statistical significance for this study was taken at $p=<0.05$ level for the univariate analysis and $p=<0.01$ for the multivariate analysis.

Results:
Five predictors of the likelihood of a child being on the SNR were identified:
- social deprivation (using Townsend-Jarman indices)
- maternal medication during pregnancy
- intrauterine growth retardation (IUGR)
- congenital abnormality
- preterm delivery.

The individual predictors were also associated with the prediction of specific disabilities in the child, such as epilepsy, specific developmental delays, cerebral palsy, central nervous system abnormality, and both physical function problems (with for example mobility, feeding or dressing) and central function problems (with speech, hearing or communication).

Suggestions for further research:
Detailed behavioural evaluation of at risk groups.
Prospective study of maternal medication in pregnancy.
Research in to IUGR.

Publications:
James, D. J., Blair, M., Wilcox, M., Telfer, F., Chilvers, C., Keating, N. (March 1996). *Pregnancy risk factors for learning disability in childhood.* Final report for the Trent Regional Health Authority. Nottingham, Trent Regional Health Authority.
James, D. J., Blair, M., Wilcox, M., Telfer, F., Chilvers, C., Keating, N. (In preparation) 'Learning disorders in childhood and risk in pregnancy'.

368. PREGNANT WOMEN'S AND HEALTH CARE PROFESSIONALS' PERCEPTIONS OF RISKS DURING NORMAL PREGNANCY

January 1995–January 1998

M. Henriksen, PhD Research Student, Dr. B. Heyman, Reader in Health Sciences, Professor S. Procter, Chair of Nursing, Professor D. Watson, Head of the Institute of Health Sciences, Northumbria University. **Contact:** Mette Henriksen, Institute of Health Sciences, Northumbria University at Newcastle, Coach Lane Campus, Newcastle NE7 7XA. Tel: (0191) 227 3024 Fax: (0191) 227 3026.

Funded as integral/additional part of a job by employer: Northern and Yorkshire Regional Health Authority.

Keywords: DECISION MAKING, EXPERIENCE (WOMEN'S), GROUNDED THEORY, HEALTH BELIEFS, MIDWIVES' ATTITUDES, PERCEPTIONS

Aims of the study:

1. To explore the ways in which women experiencing normal pregnancy conceptualize, understand and respond to potential risks associated with their pregnancy.
2. To investigate how pregnant women account for their decisions about possible risks in pregnancy.
3. To explore how health professionals understand, manage and communicate risk information regarding prenatal testing to pregnant women.
4. To examine how pregnant women perceive and manage risk information given during prenatal genetic counselling.
5. To compare pregnant women's and health professionals' perceptions of risks involved in being 'old' and 'young' whilst pregnant.

Ethics committee approval gained:

Yes

Research design:

Qualitative and quantitative, survey.

Data Collection:

Techniques used:

Phase 1: In depth and semi-structured interviews

Phase 2: Recording of prenatal genetic counselling sessions
Individual follow up interviews with the counselled women and the prenatal counsellors

Phase 3: Content analysis of obstetric notes

Phase 4: Questionnaire

Time data were collected:

Phase 1: March 1995–December 1995

Phase 2: January 1996–September 1996

Phase 3: January 1996–September 1996

Phase 4: August 1996–August 1997

Testing of any tools used:

From the data analysed in phases 1, 2 and 3 it appeared that maternity services were being offered to women according to their age. For example the 'old' were routinely offered genetic screening, and the 'very young' were routinely offered terminations of pregnancy and support from social workers. The types of services offered to the women had profound effects on their perceptions of risks. The questionnaire designed for phase 4 was based on this information, to explore further how maternity services are allocated by professionals and how pregnant women respond to such allocations in terms of their uptake of services. Four separate pilot studies of this questionnaire were carried out prior to developing the final version.

Topics covered:

Perceptions of risk in relation to what respondents perceived as being 'too old' or 'too young' to become a mother
Communication of risk information by health care professionals and interpretation by pregnant women
Decision making regarding prenatal testing
Risk management during pregnancy
Demographic details, obstetric and medical history

Setting for data collection:

Pregnant women's homes, antenatal clinic.

Details about sample studied:
Planned size of sample:

Phase 1: 48 pregnant women
Phase 2: 18 counselling sessions. Up to 40 follow up interviews with the women. Up to nine follow up interviews with the counsellors.
Phase 3: 250 sets of obstetric notes
Phase 4: 2000 questionnaires.

Rationale for planned size:

Phase 1: Theoretical sampling – sampled until saturation.
Phase 2: To include all the counsellors at the study hospital, and women at three separate stages of decision making (after counselling and before testing; after testing and before results known; after results known).
Phase 3: Stratified sampling according to maternal age.
Phase 4: All pregnant women over 34 weeks gestation attending the antenatal clinic during six months.

Entry criteria:

Phase 1: Included women having a 'normal' pregnancy; excluded women with a complicated obstetric or medical history.
Phase 2: All prenatal genetic counsellors working at the study hospital. Women receiving genetic counselling for advanced maternal age.
Phase 3: Obstetric notes of women over 34 weeks gestation.
Phase 4: Pregnant women over 34 weeks gestation attending the antenatal clinic.

Sample selection:

Phase 1: Theoretical sampling – sampled until saturation.
Phase 2: Total population of genetic counsellors. Convenience sample of women.
Phase 3: Stratified according to maternal age.
Phase 4: Total sample over six months.

Actual sample size:
As planned

Response rate:
Phase 1: 48 in depth interviews with pregnant women have been carried out.

Phase 2: 16 genetic counselling sessions were recorded (89 per cent). Eleven of these women (69 per cent) had follow up interviews. Of the six women (55 per cent) who chose amniocentesis, four had three follow up interviews and two had one. Both women (18 per cent) who chose AFP testing had three follow up interviews. Of the three women (27 per cent) who chose to have no testing, one was followed up once and two twice.

Number of follow up interviews: 24 (60 per cent).

Interviewing of the counsellors is in progress.

Phase 3: 100 per cent.

Phase 4: 500 completed questionnaires have been returned to date (100 per cent interim response rate).

Interventions, Outcomes and Analysis:
Analysis:
Phases 1&2: Using a grounded theory approach the constant comparison analysis techniques will be used, aided by NUDIST (Non-Numerical Unstructured Data Indexing, Searching and Theory building package).

Phase 3: Content analysis, using the SPSS software package.

Phase 4: SPSS for quantitative data, manual indexing for qualitative data.

Results:
In Phase 1, a grounded theory approach to data collection and analysis has been used. Age emerged as a major construct for women in the context of pregnancy. Two major categories emerged from the data; the social construction of age as a risk factor in pregnancy, and the management of decisions about 'age related' screening tests.

The notion of being old versus young involves a binary categorization of the continuous quality of age. In classifying themselves as 'old' or 'young', women had to decide where the boundary lay. Judgements varied but were bound up with the perceived need to have genetic tests. Women used age, reduced to a binary category with variable cutoff points, to determine their eligibility for genetic testing. The women undertook a form of cost benefit analysis in which they first decided whether they might be willing to have a termination. They considered not only the outcomes they wanted for the baby, but also the implications for the wider family relationships and their own capacity to cope. In their appraisal of the risks involved in the various choices, women used induction from specific experiences more frequently than codified forms of abstract knowledge.

Results from Phases 2–4 are in preparation.

Heyman, B., Henriksen, M. (1997). 'The management of Health Risks'. In: Heyman, B. (Ed.) *Risk, Health and Health Care: A Critical Approach.* (Chapter 2) London: Edward Arnold Publications. *(In press)*

Henriksen, M., Heyman, B. (1997). 'Being "Old" and Pregnant'. In: Heyman, B. (Ed) *Risk, Health and Health Care: A Critical Approach.* (Chapter 7) London: Edward Arnold Publications. *(In press)*

429. OBSTETRICIANS' VIEWS ON PRENATAL SCREENING AND DIAGNOSIS

January 1993–September 1993

J. M. Green. **Contact:** J. M. Green, Senior Lecturer, Midwifery Studies, University of Leeds, 22 Hyde Terrace, Leeds LS2 9LN. Tel: (0113) 233 6888. Fax: (0113) 244 9730.

Funded as part of a job by a Fellowship award from the Institute for Social Studies in Medical Care.

Keywords: ALPHA FETO-PROTEIN, AMNIOCENTESIS, ANTENATAL SCREENING, DOWN'S SYNDROME, FETAL ABNORMALITY, SPINA BIFIDA, TERMINATION OF PREGNANCY, TRIPLE TEST

Aims of the study:

To examine obstetricians' attitudes to prenatal screening and diagnosis, and termination of pregnancy more generally. To compare the results with those of a similar study carried out in 1980 (Farrant 1985; see Additional relevant information).

Ethics committee approval gained:

No

Research design:

Descriptive, quantitative, comparative, survey.

> **Data collection:**
> > **Techniques used:**
> > > Questionnaire
> >
> > **Time data were collected:**
> > > During 1993
> >
> > **Testing of any tools used:**
> > > Questionnaire was based on that developed by Wendy Farrant in 1980.
> >
> > **Topics covered:**
> > > Attitudes towards and resources for prenatal testing and termination of pregnancy. Demographic information.

Setting for data collection:
>Postal questionnaire

Details about sample studied:
Planned size of sample:
>323

Rationale for planned size:
>Same size as the earlier study. A large proportion of obstetricians.

Entry criteria:
Inclusions:
>Member or Fellow of RCOG, living in England or Wales.

Exclusions:
>Retired, academic appointment, not practising obstetrics, had been targeted in another recent study.

Sample selection:
>All who met the inclusion criteria and who returned the questionnaire.

Actual sample size:
>554 questionnaires were sent out.

Response rate:
>After two reminders, 393 questionnaires were returned (71 per cent). 357 (64 per cent) of these met the criteria and were analyzed.

Interventions, outcomes and analysis:
Analysis:
>Descriptive statistics.

Results:
The introduction of serum screening for Down's syndrome was a major development that occurred between the two surveys. Some form of serum screening for Down's syndrome was being offered by all but 6 per cent of respondents. Serum screening for Down's syndrome was consistently perceived as being more problematic than serum screening for neural tube defects.

Where direct comparisons with the original survey are possible, there are striking similarities, as well as some notable differences. The proportion of consultants with a conscientious objection to termination of pregnancy was very similar (9 per cent in 1980 and 10 per cent in 1993). In both surveys virtually all conscientious objectors said that they made an exception for cases of severe fetal abnormality. The proportion agreeing with the statement 'The state should not be expected to pay for the specialized care of a child with a severe handicap in cases where the parents had declined the offer of prenatal diagnosis of the handicap' was identical in the two surveys (13 per cent).

A major difference between the surveys was in the answer to the question 'Do you generally require that a patient should agree to the termination of an affected pregnancy before proceeding with amniocentesis/CVS?'. In 1980, 75 per cent answered 'Yes'; in 1993, this response was given by just 34 per cent (n=121). A related question was agreeing to prenatal diagnosis for 'a 42 year old mother of a child with Down's syndrome who was firmly opposed to the idea of abortion but had nevertheless decided that she would like to know in advance whether her next child was affected'. In 1980 over half the respondents would refuse; in 1993 only 9 per cent would refuse.

Recommendations from this study:
That obstetricians' attitudes be taken into account when considering new screening tests.

Additional relevant information:
A survey was carried out in 1980 by the Institute for Social Studies in Medical Care which examined consultant obstetricians' attitudes towards prenatal screening and diagnosis, and their attitudes towards termination of pregnancy both in the case of fetal abnormality and otherwise. This was reported in the publication below.

Farrant, W. 'Who's for amniocentesis? The politics of prenatal screening'. In: Homans, H. (Ed) (1985) *The Sexual Politics of Reproduction.* London: Gower.

Publications from this study:
Green, J. M. (1993) 'Ethics and late termination of pregnancy'. (Letter) *Lancet,* 342, p.1179.
Green, J. M. (1994). 'Serum screening for Down's syndrome: the experiences of obstetricians in England and Wales'. *British Medical Journal,* 309, pp.769–72.
Green, J. M. (1995). 'Obstetricians' views on prenatal diagnosis and termination of pregnancy: 1980 compared with 1993'. *British Journal of Obstetrics and Gynaecology,* 102, pp.228–32.
Green, J. M. (1996). 'Warning that reminders will be sent increases response rate'. *Quality and Quantity* 30(4), pp.449–50.

430. DETECTION OF FETAL ABNORMALITY AT DIFFERENT GESTATIONS: IMPACT ON PARENTS AND SERVICE IMPLICATIONS
June 1996–November 1999
J. M. Green; Helen Statham, Research Associate; Wendy Solomou, Research Associate.
Contact: J. M. Green, Senior Lecturer, Midwifery Studies, University of Leeds, 22 Hyde Terrace, Leeds LS2 9LN. Tel: (0113) 233 6888. Fax: (0113) 244 9730.

Funded as part of a job by an award form the NHS Executive (Mother and Child Health).

Keywords: ANTENATAL CARE, COMMUNICATION (INTERPROFESSIONAL), EXPERIENCE (PARENTS'), FETAL ABNORMALITY, GRIEF, INTRAPROFESSIONAL SUPPORT, STAFF ATTITUDES, SUPPORT (PROFESSIONAL), TERMINATION OF PREGNANCY

Aims of the study:

1. To investigate the experiences, views and feelings of women and their partners who have a serious abnormality confirmed at different gestations, and to compare these with women and their partners where such abnormalities are not detected until after delivery.

2. To examine the range of professional inputs that are or might be received by a couple in whom a fetal abnormality is detected and how these are coordinated. To determine to what extent these are different for abnormalities detected in early, middle or late pregnancy or after delivery.

3. To investigate the experiences, views and feelings of health professionals involved in such cases.

Ethics committee approval gained:

Yes

Research design:

Descriptive, qualitative and quantitative, comparative, survey.

Data collection:
Techniques used:

Interviews, questionnaires, diaries.

Time data were collected:

Initial letter to parents approximately three weeks after diagnosis of fetal abnormality. Interview arranged when consent form returned, approximately one month after diagnosis. Follow up contacts at one month after expected date of delivery (EDD) and at 13 months after diagnosis.

Testing of any tools used:

Questionnaires currently being piloted (September 1996).

Topics covered:

Parents:	Events leading up to diagnosis. Termination of pregnancy (if appropriate). Professional inputs and coordination afterwards.
Professionals:	Experiences, difficulties and needs in dealing with cases of fetal abnormality.

Setting for data collection:

Women's homes, postal questionnaire, staff workplaces.

Details about sample studied:
Planned size of sample:

210 women, with their partners wherever possible.

Rationale for planned size:

As large as practicable for interviews, and large enough to detect statistically significant differences between groups if these exist.

Entry criteria:

Inclusions:

Women who have a diagnosis of abnormality for which termination of pregnancy would be discussed under Ground E (serious handicap) before 24 weeks of pregnancy, at one of seven study units all in the former North West Thames Region.

Exclusions:

Women who do not speak English (it is hoped that a subsequent study will include this group).

Sample selection:

Consecutive cases from each unit that meet the study criteria, until there are seven groups of thirty women.

Actual sample size:

Not yet known.

Response rate:

Not yet known.

Interventions, outcomes and analysis:

Main outcomes measured:

Parents' emotional wellbeing, descriptive data.

Analysis:

Atlas-ti software for qualitative data. Anova software for quantitative data.

Results:

Expected in late 1999.

425. ANTENATAL HIV ANTIBODY TESTING: A SURVEY OF MATERNITY UNITS IN THE UNITED KINGDOM

November 1995–January 1996

Christine Ruby, Catherine Siney, Drug Liaison Midwife. **Contact:** Christine Ruby, Lecturer in Midwifery and Women's Health, School of Health Studies, Worcester College of Higher Education, Henwick Grove, Worcester WR2 6AJ. Tel: (01905) 855360.

Funded by the Royal College of Nursing Midwifery Society. Up to 2 hours/week of own time spent.

Keywords: ANTENATAL SCREENING, CARE COMPARISONS, HIV, HIV ANTIBODY TESTING, INFECTION, INFECTION RATES, MATERNITY SERVICES

Aims of the study:

To identify the extent and level of antenatal human immunodeficiency virus (HIV) antibody testing in the UK.

To assess the influence of the Department of Health (DOH) Guidelines on these programmes.

Ethics committee approval gained:
No. This was a survey of existing service provision.

Research design:
Descriptive, quantitative, survey.

Data collection:
Techniques used:
Self-completion questionnaire.

Time data were collected:
Between November 1 and December 31, 1995.

Testing of any tools used:
Questionnaire tested at two maternity units.

Topics covered:
- Knowledge of regional prevalence of HIV infection in pregnant women
- Testing programmes in operation
- Number of HIV tests performed and positive results obtained during preceding 12 months
- Pre- and post-test counselling: professionals providing this service, qualification held, clinical supervision in place

Setting for data collection:
Postal survey to hospitals.

Details about sample studied:
Planned size of sample:
239 units

Rationale for planned size:
All the maternity units listed in the NHS directories for England, Wales, Scotland and Northern Ireland, to obtain information on the HIV testing service across the United Kingdom.

Entry criteria:
As above

Sample selection:
Total sample

Actual sample size:
239

Response rate:
    165 (69 per cent)

Interventions, outcomes and analysis:
    Analysis:
        Simple quantitative analysis, descriptive statistics.

Results:
- There is a wide variation in the quality of antenatal HIV antibody testing services.
- Approximately half the units stated that they did not have access to the DOH Guidelines.
- All units offering routine testing based the service on DOH guidelines. Those offering selective or on request programmes frequently provided a service that fell short of good practice.
- Regional prevalence rates of HIV infection in pregnant women were only known by a minority of units.
- Knowledge of risk criteria for HIV infection was poor.
- The majority of units were unaware how many HIV tests had been performed and how many positive results obtained.
- Pre- and post-test counselling provision was variable.
- The majority of units have failed to train midwife counsellors.
- At present Genito-Urinary Medicine (GUM) clinics provide a substantial part of the pre- and post-test counselling service for pregnant women.

Recommendations from this study:
- A quality antenatal HIV antibody testing programme should be available to all women.
- The reliance on GUM clinics to provide a substantial part of this service requires further investigation.
- Maternity units should train midwives to provide pre-and post-test counselling.

Suggestions for further research:
It would be useful to repeat this survey in 3 years time to assess improvements in the service provision.

Related study:
389. HIV AND MIDWIFERY PROJECT
The abstract appears on p.99 under *Educational studies*.

381. THE EFFECTS OF EXERCISE DURING PREGNANCY
April 1993–December 1998
Jean Rankin. **Contact:** Jean Rankin, Midwifery Lecturer, Argyll and Clyde College of Nursing and Midwifery, Paisley PA2 9PN. Tel: 0141 887 9111.

Formed part of a course. Mainly self-funded, previous employer gave some study time. 6–12 hours/week of own time spent.

Keywords: ADAPTATION TO PARENTHOOD, ANTENATAL EDUCATION, BODY IMAGE, CARE COMPARISONS, EXERCISE (ANTENATAL), POSTNATAL HEALTH, PREGNANCY, SELF ESTEEM

Aims of the study:
The study hypothesises that:
Women who undertake an exercise programme during pregnancy will demonstrate:
1. Significantly improved psychological and physical well being;
2. Significantly more positive adjustments and attitudes to the pregnancy than women in the control group.

Ethics committee approval gained:
Yes

Research design:
Experimental, qualitative, randomized controlled trial.

Data Collection:
Techniques used:
Interviews, questionnaires, case note review and record of physical activity.

Time data were collected:
1. 12–16 weeks gestation
2. 36–40 weeks gestation
3. 12–16 weeks postnatally

Testing of any tools used:
Questionnaires used are well validated. Semi-structured interview was for pilot study only. Changes were made to the methodology of the main study based on findings from the pilot study.

Topics covered:
Psychological and physical well being
Attitudes and adaptations to pregnancy
Birth outcome
Postnatal well being

Setting for data collection:
Hospital and community settings.

Details about sample studied:
Planned size of sample:
30–50 exercise group; 30–50 control group.

Rationale for planned size:
Methodology discussed with statistician. Test and power of tests taken into consideration. Estimated sample size given.

Entry criteria:
Inclusion:
> Primigravid; singleton pregnancy; no history of any medical problems; identified as 'Midwifery care' by consultant obstetrician.

Sample selection:
> Random

Actual sample size:
> Not yet known.

Interventions, Outcomes and Analysis:
Interventions used:
> The antenatal and postnatal exercise programme offered to the experimental group includes a range of activities such as cycling, walking, swimming and aquanatal as well as structured exercise classes, in addition to the existing antenatal education programme. The control group received standard care.

Main outcomes measured:
> Physical well being; self esteem; body image; somatic symptoms; marital relationship; attitudes to pregnancy/baby; postnatal psychological well being; birth outcomes.

Analysis:
> Repeated measures analysis of variance on each variable, with follow up Bonferroni based multiple comparisons. Minitab statistical package.

Results:
Expected 1998.

209. EVALUATION OF A NEW PARENTHOOD PROGRAMME AVAILABLE FOR PRIMIGRAVIDAE

January 1993–September 1996

Norma Aikman, Tricia Murphy-Black. **Contact:** Norma Aikman, Parenthood Department, Simpson Memorial Maternity Pavilion, Lauriston Place, Edinburgh, EH3 9EF. Tel: (0131) 536 4290.

Funded as integral/additional part of a job by employer: Health Board. 2–6 hours/week of own time spent.

Keywords: CONSUMER LED EDUCATION, CONSUMER SATISFACTION, EDUCATION FOR PARENTHOOD, MIDWIFERY EDUCATION (CURRICULUM), PRIMIGRAVIDAE

Aims of the study:

Following a survey at the study hospital in 1990, a new programme of parenthood sessions was introduced in February 1992. As recommended in the 1990 survey, this new programme actively involved clients in determining the content of sessions, and used a greater variety of teaching and learning methods. The study abstracted here sought to identify the outcome of these changes.

Ethics committee approval gained:

Yes

Research design:

Descriptive, qualitative, quantitative, survey.

Data Collection
Techniques used:

Questionnaires.

Time data were collected:

On completion of the Parenthood Programme (prenatal group 1) and within 48 hours of delivery (postnatal group 2).

Testing of any tools used:

Pre-testing and pilot study was undertaken with 30 primigravid women, 15 prenatal and 15 postnatal, in November 1992.

Topics covered:

Parenthood Programme for primigravidae

Setting for data collection:

Urban hospital.

Details about sample studied:
Planned size of sample:

500 (200 prenatal, 300 postnatal).

Rationale for planned size:

To ensure that less motivated clients who did not complete the Parenthood Programme are included in the postnatal sample.

Entry criteria:

Exclusion:

Within the postnatal group mothers of a sick baby or stillbirth; medically unfit women.

Sample selection:

Convenience sample.

Actual sample size:

500 (200 prenatal, 300 postnatal).

Interventions, Outcomes and Analysis:
Analysis:
Data coded and verified. Analysis involved cross tabulations of obstetric and demographic data with data about preparation and/ or Parenthood Programme sessions.

Results:
Evaluations of the Parenthood Programme sessions were generally favourable. The mean scores demonstrated an overall satisfaction with the new programme, although the sessions focusing on labour had slightly higher mean scores than those on early pregnancy. All methods of teaching were found to be helpful, and 421 women (85.6 per cent) said the sessions were pitched at a level they could understand. Lectures and demonstrations, the more formal approach to information giving, were rated highest, whilst buzz groups and games received a lower rating. 45.2 per cent of the women gave further positive comments, with 20.7 per cent volunteering that they had felt prepared for the birth.

Recommendations from this study:
Organizational change to introduce team care has meant it is not possible to make recommendations based on this study.

Suggestions for further research:
This study should be replicated once the change to team care has been completed.

394. SIBLING PREPARATION FOR THE ARRIVAL OF THE NEW BABY
July 1994–March 1995
Bibi Shairoon Kelsall, Midwife Teacher (retired). **Contact:** Mrs Bibi S. Kelsall, via MIRIAD office.

Funded by the researcher as part of a BSc course. 2–6 hours per week of own time spent.

Keywords: ADAPTATION TO PARENTHOOD, ANTENATAL BOOKING INTERVIEW, ANTENATAL EDUCATION, BONDING, BREASTFEEDING, ETHNIC GROUPS, FAMILIES, PERCEPTIONS OF PARENTHOOD (WOMEN'S)

Aims of the study:
To establish the extent of current antenatal preparation of siblings by parents or during parenthood preparation classes. To find out whether mothers-to-be who already have one or more children would like sibling preparation classes to be introduced.

Ethics committee approval gained:
Yes

Research design:
Descriptive, quantitative, survey.

Data collection:
Techniques used:
Questionnaires.

Time data were collected:
At the antenatal booking visit.

Testing of any tools used:
During the 8 week pilot study 50 questionnaires were distributed to multigravid women at their antenatal booking visit. Nine completed questionnaires were returned.

Topics covered:
Preparation parents already offer their children
Preparation parents would like for their children
Ages of existing children
Behavioural problems regarding new siblings
Educational qualifications and ages of parents
Response to proposed sibling preparation classes by socio-economic and ethnic group

Setting for data collection:
Hospital, health centres and women's homes in an urban setting.

Details about sample studied:
Planned size of sample:
75 questionnaires for main study.

Rationale for planned size:
Convenience.

Entry criteria:
Inclusions:
Multigravid women attending antenatal booking sessions during the three month study period.

Sample selection:
Convenience.

Actual sample size:
75 questionnaires were distributed.

Response rate:
54 completed questionnaires were returned (72 per cent). In the main study a stamped addressed envelope was included for return of the questionnaire and it is thought that this accounts for the improved response rate.

Interventions, outcomes and analysis:

Analysis:

Demographic details, closed questions with yes/no answers and listing and attitude scales were allocated coding numbers. SPSS/PC computer software package was used for analysis.

Results:

Respondents told their 2–12 year old children about the new baby during the second and third trimesters. Some told their teenage children during the first trimester. On the whole, respondents favoured the introduction of sibling preparation classes. Mothers wanted their children to see newborn babies in the hospital where their baby was to be born. Ideally, and with their parents' permission, this would include babies at the breast and babies having special care. Other wishes were to have their children see videos of childbirth, meet staff prior to the birth, be present at the birth, and be involved in the care of the new baby in the postnatal ward. There was some evidence that different socio-economic groups wanted different preparation for their children.

Recommendations from this study:

Classes for mothers and siblings could be planned to run concurrently in the same building. Parents should have the major role in deciding the content of any sibling preparation class. Midwives may have educational needs to be met before they take on the role of sibling educators.

Suggestions for further research:

Replication of the study with a larger multi-ethnic sample in a multi-centre setting. Identify midwives' attitudes to these proposed classes.

401. ARE FATHERS PREPARED FOR LABOUR? AN INVESTIGATION OF THE FATHER'S ROLE DURING CHILDBIRTH

October 1994–March 1995

Alison Powell. **Contact:** Alison Powell, Midwife/Ward Manager, Ward M2, Maternity Unit, Bradford Royal Infirmary, Duckworth Lane, Bradford, West Yorkshire BD9 6RJ. Tel: (01274) 364531.

Formed part of BHSc in Midwifery Studies. Employer gave at least 2 hours per week study time for 6 months. Otherwise self-funded. 6–12 hours/week of own time spent initially, more in the second three months.

Keywords: BIRTH PARTNER, CHILDBIRTH, EDUCATION FOR PARENTHOOD, PERCEPTIONS OF CHILDBIRTH, PERCEPTIONS OF PARENTHOOD (FATHERS'), PERCEPTIONS OF PARENTHOOD (MOTHERS'), PERCEPTIONS OF PARENTHOOD (MIDWIVES'), PRIMIGRAVIDAE

Aims of the study:

Study question: What is the father's role during labour and delivery, and how does he need to be prepared and supported to fulfil that role?

Study aims:
- To establish the role expected of the father in labour and delivery by fathers, mothers and midwives, using the framework of roles identified by Chapman (1991).
- To elicit the main activities embarked upon by fathers to support/assist their partners during labour and delivery.
- To ascertain fathers' sources of information, and which they find most useful as preparation for childbirth.
- To highlight contributions of midwives which have helped fathers to meet their expectations of themselves as birth partners.

Ethics committee approval gained:

Yes

Research design:

Survey. The feasibility study included some quantitative data. The main study was a qualitative, descriptive study.

Data collection:
Techniques used:
Semistructured joint interviews with couples, recording the perspectives of both mothers and fathers.
Questionnaire sent to midwives attending the births.

Time data were collected:
Couples interviewed during the mothers' postnatal hospital stay.
Questionnaire sent to the midwife before the couple were interviewed.

Testing of any tools used:
Feasibility study looked at one month's delivery records and found that 81.5 per cent of British fathers and 58 per cent of Pakistani fathers were present at the birth of their babies.
Interview schedule piloted with 5 couples and questionnaire piloted with 9 midwives.

Topics covered:
- Childbirth expectations and experience
- Parentcraft preparation – sources of information
- Father's role in labour
- Support – perceptions of fathers, mothers and midwives

Setting for data collection:
Urban hospital maternity unit

Details about sample studied:
Planned size of sample:
10 couples and 30 midwives

Rationale for planned size:
Couples – realistic sample for a qualitative study in the time available.
Midwives – the whole group available from delivery suite.

Entry criteria:
Inclusions:
Couples who had both become parents for the first time, who could hold a conversation in English and consented to take part in the study. All midwives allocated to Delivery Suite during the study period.

Exclusions:
Mother or baby unwell. Couples whose baby was born by elective caesarean section. Couples whose baby had died. No midwives were excluded.

Sample selection:
Convenience sample of mothers; whole group of delivery suite midwives.

Actual sample size:
10 couples and 30 midwives.

Response rate:
Couples 100 per cent, midwives 90 per cent (27 usable returns).

Interventions, outcomes and analysis:
Analysis:
Content analysis used to identify key words and phrases and common themes which were then built into categories and discussed.

Results:
- The major component of the father's role during childbirth was seen as 'support', encompassing emotional, verbal and physical helping activities. Mothers considered communication to be a vital role for fathers assisting in childbirth. Couples perceived this as a supportive role, whereas midwives saw it as advocacy.
- Fathers considered practical involvement important. All fathers in the study undertook some form of supportive practical task.
- Antenatal information and preparation for labour was sought by all the fathers to varying degrees. Books and leaflets were their primary source of information.
- All the fathers in the study considered continuity of midwifery carer in labour to be an important issue.

Recommendations from this study:

In spite of the high proportion of fathers attending births, there is a dearth of information about their needs and experiences. This small exploratory study has identified some areas which could be explored in a larger study.

Suggestions for further research:

Why do some women labour with no support from a birth partner?
Are there specific cultural influences on the involvement of fathers in childbirth?

Clinical studies: birth and after

350. THE USE OF TRANSCUTANEOUS NERVE STIMULATION (TENS) IN LABOUR: A STUDY TO ASCERTAIN THE OPTIMUM TIME FOR COMMENCING TENS

August 1995–January 1997

Ian Swain, Terri Coates, Peter Kelly, Pippa Swayne. **Contact:** Terri Coates, Research Midwife, Department of Medical Physics and Biomedical Engineering, Salisbury District Hospital, Odstock, Salisbury, Wiltshire SP2 8BJ. Tel: (017222) 336262, Ext. 4065. Fax: (017222) 337272, Ext. 4064.

Funded as integral/additional part of a job by funding agency: RAYMAR – Business sponsor. TENS machines are among the products which RAYMAR market. The company has no control over the research or future publications. 6–12 hours/week of own time spent.

Keywords: PAIN, PAIN ASSESSMENT, PAIN RELIEF (LABOUR), PAIN RELIEF (PRESCRIBING), TENS

Aims of the study:

To ascertain the optimum time to commence the use of TENS for pain control in labour.

Ethics committee approval gained:

Yes

Research design:

Qualitative, quantitative.

Data Collection:
Techniques used:

Questionnaires, case note review.

Time data were collected:

Prior to labour, during labour and as soon as practicable after labour.

Testing of any tools used:

Questionnaires were tested/piloted.
An established pain scoring system was used.
A fourth group of 30 women has been added to increase the amount and reliability of data on the pain score itself. This is a convenience sample of women admitted to labour ward in labour who complete a pain score but do not use TENS.

Topics covered:

Use of TENS
TENS for pain control in labour
Pain control in labour

Setting for data collection:
Hospital, client's home if having a home birth.

Details about sample studied:
Planned size of sample:
Originally 60 women, 20 in each of three groups. Because pain scores were not being filled in on Labour Ward for about one third of women, the sample size was increased to 90 women, 30 in each group, in an attempt to reach the size originally planned.

Rationale for planned size:
Advised that this sample size would give statistically meaningful results. Thought to be achievable in six months, but recruitment has been slow.

Entry criteria:
Inclusion:
Client self referral to TENS group.

Exclusion:
Women with pacemakers.

Sample selection:
Convenience

Actual sample size:
Last women recruited to the trial are due to give birth by mid-August 1996.

Interventions, Outcomes and Analysis:
Interventions used:
Group 1 – TENS used from 37 weeks gestation for two hrs/day.
Group 2 – TENS used in early labour at home.
Group 3 – TENS used from admission to labour ward.
Group 4 – Control group. 30 consecutive admissions to labour ward in established labour, any type of pain control.

Main outcomes measured:
Women's use of TENS.
Women's ratings of the effectiveness of TENS.

Results:
Not yet completed.

Additional relevant information:
Recruitment to the trial has been slow since the introduction of a birthing pool to the Labour Ward in Autumn 1995. The researcher would be interested to ask women if those who would previously have chosen to use TENS are opting instead to use the pool.

283. EPIDURAL ANALGESIA AND POSITION IN THE PASSIVE SECOND STAGE OF LABOUR: OUTCOMES FOR NULLIPAROUS WOMEN

January 1993–September 1997

Soo Downe, David Gerrett, Mary Renfrew. **Contact:** S. M. Downe, Research Midwife, Derby City General Hospital NHS Trust, Maternity and Gynaecology Research and Audit Office, 3rd Floor, Derby City General Hospital NHS Trust, Uttoxeter Road, Derby, DE22 3NE. Tel: (01332) 340131, Ext. 5070. Email: derbymatgynea@dial. pipex.com..

Formed part of a course. Funded as integral/additional part of a job by employer. SDHA Nurses and Midwives Research Funds provided additional funding. 2 hours/week of own time spent.

Keywords: APGAR SCORES, CONSUMER OPINION, EPIDURALS, EPISIOTOMY, LABOUR, OUTCOMES (MATERNAL), OUTCOMES (NEONATAL), POSITIONS (LABOUR), SECOND STAGE

Aims of the study:

1. To test the null hypothesis: The use of the lateral position in the passive second stage of labour will have no significant effect on
   a) the rate of instrumental vaginal deliveries;
   b) the rate of episiotomies;
   c) fetal Apgar;
   and neither staff nor women taking part in the trial will express a preference for either position.
2. To assess the effect of involving service users and midwives in the design of recommendations for practice based on trial results.

Ethics committee approval gained:

Yes

Research design:

Qualitative, quantitative, randomized controlled trial, survey.

Data Collection:
Techniques used:

1. Pre and post trial questionnaires to staff
2. Pre delivery questionnaires to women
3. RCT (including visual analogue pain scales)
4. Post delivery questionnaires to women at two weeks and three months postpartum.

Time data were collected:

1. One month pre-trial and one month post-trial.
2. At time of consenting.
3. During labour.
4. Two weeks and three months postpartum.

Testing of any tools used:
1. Tested with 10 midwives.
2. Pre-validated scale (Speilberger State/Trait Anxiety inventory).
3. A composite questionnaire mostly comprising established tools – tested for face validity and comprehension with 10 postnatal women.

Topics covered:
- Staff preference for position in labour
- Anxiety levels (State/Trait) – women
- Labour outcomes, intrapartum pain levels and a range of demographic details
- Maternal confidence and self image, maternal morbidity, infant feeding method, labour fulfilment, anxiety, difficulty levels
- Maternal and staff reaction to results and their views on potential for implementation

Setting for data collection:
Hospital, client's home.

Details about sample studied:
Planned size of sample:
200 (100 in each group), required recruitment of 500 women antenatally.

Rationale for planned size:
Sufficient to demonstrate a 50 per cent reduction in forceps rate if it exists based on power calculation (alpha = 95 per cent, beta = 80 per cent).

Entry criteria:
Inclusion:
All nulliparous women who have consented antenatally who:
- still consent once an epidural has been sited in labour;
- are 36+ weeks gestation;
- who have a singleton pregnancy;
- cephalic presentation;
- live fetus.

Exclusion:
Intrauterine fetal death, severe maternal hypertension, severe fetal growth retardation, breech, multiple pregnancies, trial of labour, trial of uterine scar.

Sample selection:
Women entered as convenience sample then randomized.

Actual sample size:
107

Interventions, Outcomes and Analysis:
Interventions used:
The use of either the sitting or lateral position in the passive 2nd stage of labour.

Main outcomes measured:
Forceps rate; ventouse rate; perineal trauma rate; fetal Apgar; maternal morbidity; maternal impressions of labour and delivery and their role in it.

Analysis:
Using SPSS: Chi-square, t-test, Mann-Whitney U, simple frequencies and means, factor analysis and logistic regression.

Results:
Some results have been submitted for publication, others are in preparation.

239. PRELIMINARY EVALUATION OF HYDROTHERAPY IN LABOUR, USING HARD INDICATORS
December 1989–January 1994
Dianne Garland, Keith Jones. **Contact:** Dianne Garland, Senior Midwife Practice and Research, Mid Kent Health Care Trust, Maidstone Hospital, Hermitage Lane, Maidstone, Kent, ME16 9QQ. Tel: (01622) 729000, Ext. 4421. Fax: (01622) 720807.

Funded as integral/additional part of a job by employer: Maidstone Hospital.

Keywords: HYDROTHERAPY, LABOUR, WATER BIRTH

Aims of the study:
To compare three groups of women in 'normal' labour:
1. Those who did not use hydrotherapy.
2. Those who used hydrotherapy during labour but left the water prior to delivery.
3. Those who delivered in water.

Ethics committee approval gained:
No

Research design:
Descriptive, qualitative, quantitative.

Data Collection:
Techniques used:
Extraction of data from daily activity records in delivery suite.

Time data were collected:
Retrospectively.

Testing of any tools used:
No special tools used.

Topics covered:
Use of drugs
Instrumental delivery
Operative delivery
Duration of labour
Naturally occurring genital trauma
Post-partum haemorrhage

Setting for data collection:
Hospital.

Details about sample studied:
Planned size of sample:
600 (200 in each of the three groups).

Rationale for planned size:
Records of 229 waterbirths in the department were available.

Entry criteria:
Inclusion:
More than 37 weeks gestation, singleton, cephalic presentation, no known or envisaged problems.

Sample selection:
Convenience.

Actual sample size:
429

Response rate:
N/A

Interventions, Outcomes and Analysis:
Analysis:
SPSS SYSTAT.

Results:
For research purposes, waterbirth clients should be distinguished from women who immerse during the first stage of labour only.

Our waterbirth clients:
* needed no intramuscular or epidural drugs
* had a slightly increased incidence of genital tract tears but also an increased frequency of intact perineum (NB episiotomy not performed in water)
* did not have a significantly increased risk for postpartum haemorrhage
* delivered fewer babies with low Apgar scores at one minute the 'dry' birth mothers.

35

The findings may be peculiar to the data set used. The ability to generalise would depend on replication, and this is in progress.

Garland, D., Jones, K. (1994). 'Waterbirth, 'First stage' immersion or non-immersion?' *British Journal of Midwifery* 2, pp.113–20.
Garland, D. (1995). *Waterbirth – An Attitude to Care*. Hale: Books for Midwives Press.

Related study:
400. WOMEN'S EXPERIENCE OF WATERBIRTH
The abstract appears on p.72 under *Clinical studies: women's views.*

396. LABOUR PAIN, ANXIETY, LABOUR LENGTH AND LABOUR PAIN RECALL
June 1993–November 1994
Margaret Yerby. **Contact:** Margaret Yerby, Senior Lecturer in Midwifery, Wolfson Institute, Westell House, Thames Valley University, 32-38 Uxbridge Road, Ealing, London W5 2BS. Tel: (0181) 280 5081 Fax: (0181) 280 5137.

Part submission for a Masters degree. 2–6 hours per week of own time spent. Study was self-funded.

Keywords: ANXIETY, DELIVERY, LABOUR (DURATION), PAIN, PAIN ASSESSMENT, PAIN EXPERIENCE, PRIMIGRAVIDAE.

Aims of the study:
To investigate the hypothesis:
Women who have longer labours will be more anxious and have more pain intensity, and will recall their labours with more pain intensity and more pain distress.

Ethics committee approval gained:
Yes

Research design:
A matched subjects design in three phases of pregnancy, using quantitative data and focusing on relationships between variables.

    Data collection:
        Techniques used:
            Three stage questionnaire and information about the delivery from computer records and notes.

        Time data were collected:
            Questionnaire at 20+ weeks of pregnancy, at diagnosis of labour and during the first 24 hours after the birth.

Testing of any tools used:
Used established tools; Spielberger's anxiety inventory (state and trait), and a visual analogue scale of 1–10 for intensity and distress of pain.

Topics covered:
Anxiety scores before, during and after labour; pain scores (both intensity and distress) during and after labour; length of labour; recall of labour pain intensity, distress and coping.

Setting for data collection:
An urban teaching hospital.

Details about sample studied:
Planned size of sample:
150

Rationale for planned size:
Convenience

Entry criteria:
Inclusions:
Women aged 20–40, having a first, healthy, singleton pregnancy, a spontaneous labour at 37–42 weeks, and a vaginal delivery of a live baby.

Exclusions:
Women suffering chronic pain, e.g. back pain, arthritis; history of treatment for infertility; antepartum haemorrhage, pregnancy induced hypertension, pre-term labour, antenatal admission to hospital prior to labour.

Sample selection:
Convenience. The parent education midwife explained the study at hospital parent education classes and volunteers from the classes formed the sample.

Actual sample size:
140

Response rate:
70 were returned, 32 (22 per cent) were complete and these were analysed.

Interventions, outcomes and analysis:
Analysis:
SPSS computer package.

Results:
Labour length showed no significance to any of the variables and this was consistent with other research (Burns 1976, Bonnel and Boureau 1985). Correlational analysis showed that labour pain intensity to anxiety tended to significance whereas pain distress showed a positive relationship to anxiety levels at 0.01 level of significance. Postnatally women with high anxiety levels tended to recall pain with more distress; this was of borderline significance. Pain distress seemed to be an important variable in this study and an area to be pursued in further research.

Suggestions for further research:
The final sample was small and there is a need for further research in this area for midwives to improve practice and client satisfaction. A much larger sample, a research approach including both qualitative and quantitative aspects, and data on methods of pain relief used, would give more indications for practice and quality of care.

409. EMERGENCY OBSTETRIC PROCEDURES IN THE INTRAPARTUM PERIOD: A POST TRAUMATIC STRESS PERSPECTIVE

May 1994–May 1995
Angela Benbow. **Contact:** Angela Benbow, Midwife, RCOG Audit Unit, Saint Mary's Hospital, Hathersage Road, Whitworth Park, Manchester M13 0JH. Tel: (0161) 276 6300. Fax: (0161) 276 6311.

Formed part of a degree course funded by a Local Education Authority grant; the researcher also worked in clinical practice. More than 20 hours/week spent.

Keywords: ADAPTATION TO MOTHERHOOD, ANXIETY (MATERNAL), CAESAREAN SECTION, DEPRESSION, PERCEPTIONS OF CHILDBIRTH (WOMEN'S), POSTNATAL SUPPORT, PSYCHOLOGY, STRESS (MATERNAL).

Aims of the study:
To investigate the hypothesis that:
Women who undergo emergency obstetric episodes during the intrapartum period can experience a stress reaction of sufficient severity to fulfil the diagnostic criteria for Post Traumatic Stress Disorder (PTSD), as defined by the Diagnostic Statistical Manual (Fourth Edition) of the American Psychiatric Association (DSM-IV APA).

Ethics committee approval gained:
Yes

Research design:
Descriptive, qualitative and quantitative, survey of two groups.

Data collection:
Techniques used:
Questionnaire and self-report Impact of Events Scale (IES).

Time data were collected:

From women at two and at six weeks after birth, during November 1994–January 1995.

Testing of any tools used:

Used an established tool, the IES, developed by Horowitz, Wilner & Alvarez (1979) specifically to measure subjective stress.

Topics covered:

Stress (psychological/social/biological) during pregnancy, the intrapartum period, and postnatally. Occurrence of any of the obstetric episodes specified in the study. Partner's psychosocial reactions to fatherhood.

Setting for data collection:

Two postnatal wards at a single maternity unit, based on the site of a District General Hospital.

Details about sample studied:
Planned size of sample:

60 women, 30 in each group.

Rationale for planned size:

Advice from supervisors.

Entry criteria:
Inclusions:

Both groups: Women who gave birth to a live healthy baby born after at least 35 weeks of pregnancy.

Group A: Women who in addition had one or more of the following adverse episodes in the peripartum period; severe haemorrhage (antepartum, intrapartum or postpartum), intrapartum emergency caesarean section, instrumental delivery.

Group B: Women who delivered spontaneously with or without an episiotomy, the fetus presenting by the vertex.

Sample selection:

Women who fulfilled the research criteria were initially identified from the ward records and then from the casenotes. With permission from staff the researcher approached women on the ward to discuss the study. Those who fulfilled the criteria for Group A were not approached for at least 24 hours following delivery.

Actual sample size:

Group A=30. Group B=23. Total 53.

Response rate:

First survey: Group A: 25 responded (83 per cent)
                       Group B: 16 responded (70 per cent)
Second survey: Group A: 25 responded (100 per cent)
                       Group B: 16 responded (100 per cent)

Interventions, outcomes and analysis:
Main outcomes measured:

Stress reaction, defined by measuring the levels of intrusion and avoidance experienced.

Analysis:

Qualitative analyses of the comments made by the women on the questionnaire and quantitative analyses of the IES scores as follows: Two tailed *t* test for paired samples at p=0.05 using the Superstat package.

Results:

The study hypothesis was met. The women who experienced emergency obstetric episodes were more likely to demonstrate higher levels of subjective stress than the women who experienced normal deliveries. Nevertheless, some women who experienced normal deliveries did demonstrate high stress on the IES. The levels of stress demonstrated were sufficient to fulfil the criteria for PTSD. The differences between the two groups did not reach statistical significance.

However, the IES was designed to look at the effects of stressful life events on individuals. The results showed that eight women (20 per cent of the 41 respondents, six (24 per cent) from Group A and two (13 per cent) from Group B) who demonstrated high scores at six weeks had in fact increased their total IES from the two week administration, indicating abnormal stress reaction sequelae.

Recommendations from this study:

The signs and symptoms of stress reaction sequelae need to be clearly defined so that they can be more readily recognised by those caring for mothers and families.

Suggestions for further research:

A larger study with more respondents over a wider geographical area, including interviews, to consider how a stress reaction manifests itself following the birth of a baby. Analysis of available research instruments may identify some more appropriate for use in this area. Although the IES is recognised as a versatile and well standardised research tool in the field of traumatic stress, the area of childbirth may require a more specific instrument.

370. THE RANDOMIZED CONTROLLED TRIAL OF CARE OF THE PERINEUM AT DELIVERY – HANDS ON OR POISED? THE HOOP STUDY

June 1994–December 1997

Jo Garcia, Diana Elbourne, Mary Renfrew, Georgina Berridge, Ursula Bowler, Sara Bowler, Natalie Kenney, Pat Marshall, Rona McCandlish, Siobhan Scanlen, Hedwig Van Asten, Eileen Jolly, Lesley Sames, Anna Hughes, Cathy Winter, Walter Hannah, Sue McDonald, Jennifer Sleep. **Contact:** Rona McCandlish, Research Midwife, National Perinatal Epidemiology Unit, Radcliffe Infirmary, Oxford OX2 6HE. Tel: (01865) 224332. Fax: (01865) 792270. EMail: rona.mccandlish@perinatal-epidemiology.oxford.ac.uk

Funded as integral/additional part of a job by funding agency: Medical Research Council, 20 Park Crescent, London W1N 4AL.

Keywords: DELIVERY, LABOUR, MIDWIVES' CARE, OUTCOMES (PERINATAL), OUTCOMES (PERINEAL), PAIN RELIEF (PERINEUM), PERINEAL PAIN

Aims of the study:

The purpose of this trial is to compare the effects of two techniques for spontaneous delivery.

1. The midwife's hands are used to put pressure on the baby's head in the belief that flexion will be increased, and to 'guard' the perineum, and to use lateral flexion to facilitate the birth of the shoulders.
2. The midwife keeps her hands poised, prepared to put light pressure on the baby's head in case of rapid expulsion, but not to touch the head or the perineum or the shoulders otherwise.

The primary outcome to be assessed is perineal/vaginal/labial pain as reported by women who participate at ten days after birth.

Ethics committee approval gained:

Yes

Research design:

Clinical study, experimental, qualitative, quantitative, randomized controlled trial.

Data Collection:
Techniques used:
Questionnaires, labour ward register.

Time data were collected:
During labour; immediately after delivery; two days after birth; 9–11 days after birth; three months after birth.

Testing of any tools used:

Questionnaires tested by women who gave birth in Brighton during August 1994 and by midwives offering care to women who gave birth in Brighton during August 1994.

Topics covered:

Socio-demographic details
Obstetric history
Current labour outcomes (mothers and infants)
Physical and psychological outcomes (mothers)
Infant feeding
Infant physical health

Setting for data collection:

Hospital, client's home.

Details about sample studied:

Planned size of sample:

Initially, 8,500 women. The data were reviewed by the Data Monitoring Committee in August 1995, and in the light of the Committee's recommendations the planned sample size was amended to 5,500 women.

Rationale for planned size:

The original sample size was calculated using previous estimates of the incidence of perineal pain at 10 days after birth (Sleep et al 1984) to detect a 10 per cent difference in pain with 80 per cent certainty (alpha=0.05). These estimates were reviewed in the light of the interim analysis and it has been calculated that the smaller sample size will allow identification of a 10 per cent difference, if one exists.

Entry criteria:

Inclusion:

Singleton pregnancy; live fetus; cephalic presentation; gestation 37 weeks or more; spontaneous vaginal delivery considered imminent; woman willing to participate.

Exclusion:

Intrauterine death; multiple pregnancy; non-cephalic presentation; <37 weeks gestation; non vaginal/instrumental delivery planned; episiotomy prescribed; birth in water planned; woman does not wish to participate.

Sample selection:

Random

Actual sample size:

5400

Interventions, Outcomes and Analysis:
> **Interventions used:**
>> Two techniques for managing the perineum at the end of the second stage of labour:
>> 1. 'Hands On'.
>> 2. 'Hands Poised' as described under Aims of the study.

> **Main outcomes measured:**
>> Perineal/vaginal/labial pain as reported at ten days after birth by women who take part.

> **Analysis:**
>> Primary analysis by intention to treat. Secondary analyses will include stratification by centre, parity and other factors. Economic implications will be analysed.

> **Additional relevant information:**
>> Analysis and reporting are under way (June 1997).

398. DIFFERENCES IN PERINEAL TRAUMA BETWEEN BENGALI AND CAUCASIAN WOMEN
September 1993–September 1994
Priscilla Bennett. **Contact:** Priscilla Bennett, Midwife, via MIRIAD office.

Formed part of MSc course. Partly funded by the Hospital Savings Association. Over 20 hours per week of own time spent.

Keywords: ETHNIC GROUPS, PERINEAL TRAUMA, PRIMIPARAE

Aims of the study:
To compare perineal trauma between two ethnic groups to see if a difference exists. The null hypothesis postulates: There is no relationship between ethnic group and perineal trauma sustained at delivery in young primiparous women.

This was measured by comparing perineal trauma in Bengali and Caucasian women, after spontaneous birth at term of a healthy baby presenting in a vertex position, attended by a midwife or student midwife.

Ethics committee approval gained:
Yes

Research design:
Descriptive, quantitative, retrospective, survey.

> **Data collection:**
>> **Techniques used:**
>>> Case note review

Time data were collected:

Deliveries between March 1993 and January 1994 were examined retrospectively.

Testing of any tools used:

A data collection sheet was tested to ensure the information required was available in the notes.

Topics covered:

Age, height, last known pregnant weight, parity, gestation, attending midwife/student midwife, length of labour, early decelerations, analgesia, epidural anaesthesia, birth weight, neonatal head circumference.

Setting for data collection:

Inner city teaching hospital.

Details about sample studied:
Planned size of sample:

100 Bengali women and 100 Caucasian women.

Rationale for planned size:

1993 figures for perineal trauma within the study hospital revealed a 54.9 per cent perineal trauma rate. Power analysis showed that in order to observe a 20 per cent difference in the rate of perineal trauma (60–40 per cent) at the 5 per cent significance level with a power of 80 per cent, 97 women would be required in each group.

Entry criteria:
Inclusions:

Bengali and Caucasian women aged 18–30 years, having a first baby (those with one previous pregnancy loss or termination prior to 12 weeks gestation were included), a spontaneous vertex delivery between 37 and 42 weeks gestation, no signs of fetal distress, Apgar scores of 8 or more, birthweight between 2500g and 4000g, and delivered by a midwife or student midwife.

Sample selection:

Records of the first 100 women in each of the ethnic groups who gave birth after 1 March 1993 and met the selection criteria were included.

Actual sample size:

100 Bengali women and 100 white Caucasian women.

Response rate:

100 per cent

Interventions, outcomes and analysis:
    Analysis:
        Statistical Package for the Social Sciences (SPSS) was used.
        Parametric tests: Student t test, Pearson correlation coefficient test.
        Non-parametric tests: Mann-Whitney U test, chi square, Spearman
        rank correlation coefficient.

Results:
The results showed that the Bengali women had significantly more perineal trauma than the Caucasian women ($r = -0.1492$, $p<0.05$). There was no difference in episiotomy rates. The Bengali women were also significantly younger, shorter, lighter, had a shorter gestation and gave birth to lighter babies with a smaller head circumference than the Caucasian women. Of these factors only height was found to be related to perineal trauma ($r = -0.1492$, $p<0.025$). The shorter the woman, the more likely she was to sustain perineal trauma. The Bengali women had less perineal trauma when delivered by a student midwife when compared with midwife deliveries ($p<0.05$). This difference was not found amongst the white Caucasian women.

Suggestions for further research:
To examine other variables which could account for the differences in perineal trauma that have been found. A prospective study would be beneficial in order to provide more accurate data and to include the variables of language and management of labour.

Additional relevant information:
The researcher would like to acknowledge her supervisors, Ruth Bennett and Jennifer Sleep.

235. THE HINCHINGBROOKE THIRD STAGE TRIAL
June 1993–June 1996
Jane Rogers, Juliet Wood, Diana Elbourne, Rona McCandlish, Ann Truesdale. **Contact:** Jane Rogers and Juliet Wood, Midwives, Hinchingbrooke Hospital, Huntingdon, Cambs PE18 8NT. Tel: (01480) 416416 Ext. 6445. Fax: (01480) 416248.

Funded as integral/additional part of a job by funding agency: Public Health and Operational Research Award, East Anglia Regional Health Authority.

Keywords: ACTIVE MANAGEMENT, MATERNAL MORBIDITY, NEONATAL MORBIDITY, POSTPARTUM HAEMORRHAGE, THIRD STAGE

Aims of the study:
To determine whether in terms of maternal and neonatal morbidity, it is justifiable to continue with the current option of employing expectant rather than active management of the third stage of labour for women considered to be at low risk of postpartum haemorrhage (PPH) in a setting in which both managements are commonly practised. The primary hypothesis is that the active management of the third stage of labour reduces the incidence of postpartum haemorrhage, even in a setting in which both expectant and active management are routinely practised for women thought to be at low risk of postpartum haemorrhage.

Ethics committee approval gained:
Yes

Research design:
Experimental, qualitative, quantitative, randomized controlled trial.

Data Collection:
Techniques used:
Questionnaires, case note review, records of observations.

Time data were collected:
Immediately after delivery, at transfer from hospital to home and at six weeks postnatally.

Testing of any tools used:
Small pilot of questionnaires prior to trial. Sample of Edinburgh Postnatal Depression Scale scores used to validate part of six week questionnaire.

Topics covered:
Obstetric and medical history
Delivery details
Management of third stage: technique, timing, manual removal of placenta, estimated blood loss, side effects and use of oxytocics
Postnatal maternal morbidity: anaemia, blood transfusion, iron therapy, evacuation of retained products of conception, positive Kleihauer test, fatigue, depression, feeding difficulties
Neonatal jaundice treated with phototherapy
Admission to SCBU
Women's and staff views of participation in the trial
Economic/resource outcomes

Setting for data collection:
Maternity Unit in District General Hospital, rural and urban surgeries and mothers' homes.

Details about sample studied:
Planned size of sample:
2000

Rationale for planned size:
To reach statistical significance.

Entry criteria:
Inclusion:
Women at low risk of post-partum haemorrhage.

Exclusion:

Placenta praevia, previous postpartum haemorrhage, antepartum haemorrhage after 20 weeks gestation, haemoglobin <10 g/dl or mean cell volume <75, multiple pregnancy, intrauterine death, epidural, parity >5, uterine fibroid, syntocinon infusion for induction/augmentation of labour, anticoagulant therapy, instrumental/operative delivery <32/40 gestation, any other circumstances where the clinician feels there are overwhelming contra-indications to any of the forms of management.

Sample selection:

All eligible mothers. With consent, randomized to one of four groups. Recruitment ongoing.

Interventions, Outcomes and Analysis:
Interventions used:

Four management groups:
1. Active management, upright position.
2. Active management, semi-recumbent position.
3. Expectant management, upright position.
4. Expectant management, semi-recumbent position.

Active management = 1ml syntometrine IM with delivery of baby, or 10iu syntocinon IM if mother is hypertensive.

Main outcomes measured:

Postpartum haemorrhage rate, estimated blood loss, Hb and MCV (32 weeks and day 2 postnatal), length of 3rd stage, manual removal of placenta, blood transfusion, maternal fatigue and depression.

Analysis:

SPSS

Results:

Secondary analysis in progress (September 1996). Intending to submit for publication early in 1997.

199. IPSWICH CHILDBIRTH STUDY
May 1992–December 1996

C. Mackrodt, B. S. Gordon, E. Fern, S. Ayers, A. Grant, A. Truesdale. **Contact:** B. Gordon, Midwifery Clinical Specialist, Directorate of Maternity and Gynaecology, The Ipswich Hospital NHS Trust, Heath Road, Ipswich, IP4 5PD. Tel: (01473) 712233. Fax: (01473) 703400.

Funded as integral/additional part of a job and by funding agencies: National Birthday Trust, Directorate of Public Health Medicine and a Locally Organized Research Scheme.

Keywords: PERINEAL HEALING, PERINEAL PAIN, PERINEAL REPAIR, PERINEUM, PUERPERIUM, SUTURES, SUTURING

Aims of the study:

1. To compare the differences in pain, comfort and healing between suturing the perineum using the standard three layer approach and using a two layer approach leaving the skin edges apposed and unsutured.
2. To compare pain, comfort and healing rates between perineal repairs using chromic catgut and polyglactin 210 (vicryl) for suturing.

Ethics committee approval gained:

Yes

Research design:

Experimental, qualitative, quantitative, randomized controlled trial.

Data Collection:
Techniques used:

Interviews, records of observations.

Time data were collected:

Postnatally: 24–48 hours, 10–14 days and 2–3 months. Recruitment completed October 1994 for both spontaneous and instrumental deliveries.

Testing of any tools used:

Tested on a small number of women.

Topics covered:

Pain
Healing
Comfort

Setting for data collection:

Hospital and community.

Details about sample studied:
Planned size of sample:

1500

Rationale for planned size:

Statistically calculated to give 95 per cent confidence interval.

Entry criteria:
Inclusion:

Normal deliveries, 1st and 2nd degree tears or episiotomies.

Exclusion:

Third degree tears.

Lacerations which did not involve perineal skin.

Sample selection:

Computerized randomization to trial groups done by National Perinatal Epidemiology Unit.

Actual sample size:

For both interventions: 1469 spontaneous deliveries and 311 instrumental deliveries.

Response rate:

99 per cent at 24–48 hours; 99 per cent at 10–14 days; 93 per cent at three months.

Interventions, outcomes and analysis:

Interventions used

1. One group to have two layer approach to perineal repair leaving skin edges apposed and unsutured.
2. One group to have perineal repair using polyglactin 210 (vicryl) for suturing.

Main outcomes measured:

Pain, healing, comfort, resumption of sexual intercourse and degree of dyspareunia, general wellbeing.

Analysis:

Ongoing stratified analyses using ORCALC.

Results:

To follow completion of analysis. Some preliminary results have been submitted for publication. The researchers hope to be able to issue results in varying formats as well as their full report by January 1997.

Additional relevant information:

Tandem study for those women having 'simple' instrumental deliveries, started June 1993. Sample size 200–300. Separately randomized.

230. THE RESOURCE IMPLICATIONS OF DIFFERENT APPROACHES TO THE MANAGEMENT OF PERINEAL TRAUMA
November 1991–December 1996

Sarah Howard, Stavros Petrou, Denise Mickell, Louise Hallam. **Contact:** Stavros Petrou, Health Economist, National Perinatal Epidemiology Unit, Radcliffe Infirmary, Oxford, OX2 6HE. Tel: (01865) 224126. Fax: (01865) 792270. email: GENERAL@ PERINAT.OX.AC.UK

Funded as integral/additional part of a job by employer: Department of Health.

Keywords: COST EFFECTIVENESS, DYSPAREUNIA, ECONOMIC EVALUATION, PAIN, PERINEAL REPAIR, SUTURE MATERIALS, SUTURING

Aims of the study:
To provide information on the cost effectiveness of preventative and treatment interventions for perineal trauma.

Ethics committee approval gained:
No

Research design:
Descriptive, secondary use of experimental data, quantitative.

Data Collection:
Techniques used:
Interviews and questionnaires. Review of any evidence on resource use from systematic reviews of randomized controlled trials.

Topics covered:
Resources involved in the process of perineal suturing, removal of sutures, resuturing and associated perineal pain.

Setting for data collection:
Hospital and community.

Details about sample studied:
Planned size of sample:
110 (100 removal of sutures, 10 resuturing).

Rationale for planned size:
Practical

Entry criteria:
Inclusion:
Any woman having stitches removed from her perineum after childbirth by a midwife based at the Ipswich Hospital.
Any woman having her perineum resutured for whatever reason, at the Ipswich Hospital.

Sample selection:
Convenience

Actual sample size:
Recruitment ongoing.

Interventions, Outcomes and Analysis:
  Interventions used:
      So far comparing:
      1. Absorbable versus non-absorbable perineal skin sutures.
      2. Continuous versus interrupted perineal sutures.
      3. Apposing the perineal skin versus suturing.

  Main outcomes measured:
      Long term pain (3 months).
      Short term pain (10 days).
      Dyspareunia at 3 months.
      Need for removal of sutures.
      Need for resuturing.

  Analysis:
      Not yet completed.

Howard, S., Mickell, D., Mugford, M., Grant, A. (1995). 'The cost effectiveness of different approaches to perineal suturing for minimizing post-partum pain'. *British Journal of Midwifery*, Vol.3, No. 11, pp.587–90, pp.603–5.

407. SELF-MEDICATION: ANOTHER STEP IN MATERNITY WARDS DISCARDING THEIR TRADITIONAL ETHOS OF ILLNESS AND PATIENTHOOD
September 1994–May 1995
Ursula Clarke. **Contact:** Ursula Clarke, Research and Development Midwife, All Saints Hospital, Chatham, Kent ME4 5NG. Tel: (01634) 407311

Formed part of a course. Course fees provided by employer. All other costs met by researcher. 12–20 hours/week of own time spent.

Keywords: ACCOUNTABILITY, CHILDBIRTH (CHOICES), CONSULTANT UNITS, HOSPITAL POLICY, HOSPITALIZATION, MIDWIFERY EDUCATION (ACCOUNTABILITY), PAIN RELIEF, PAIN RELIEF (PRESCRIBING)

Aims of the study:
To explore the attitude of mothers and staff towards self-medication.
To determine satisfaction levels with self-medication focusing primarily on analgesic requirements.

Ethics committee approval gained:
Yes

Research design:
Quasi-experiment, qualitative and quantitative, survey.

Data collection:
Techniques used:
Questionnaires, case note review

Time data were collected:
On discharge from postnatal wards

Testing of any tools used:
Pilot study with nine mothers and four midwives

Topics covered:
Mothers: Details of hospital admission, attitudes towards self-medication, demographic and delivery details.

Midwives: Attitudes towards self-medication, attitudes towards giving out medicines, demographic details.

Setting for data collection:
Hospital; consultant obstetric unit.

Details about sample studied:
Planned size of sample:
100 mothers, 50 in each group. 26 midwives.

Rationale for planned size:
The study needed to be piloted and completed within one month so as to avoid the effect of a change of staff due to rotation.

Entry criteria:
Inclusions:
Every postnatal mother on the ward was given the choice to self-medicate or not if she:
- was well enough to self-medicate
- could read and write in English
- had no history of drug abuse or psychiatric illness
- was prescribed any regular medication including analgesia.

Sample selection:
Convenience

Actual sample size:
57 mothers and 26 midwives

Response rate:
Mothers 82 per cent, midwives 92 per cent

Interventions, outcomes and analysis:
Interventions used:
One ward allowed all mothers eligible and who wished to, to self-medicate. The other ward continued to have midwives administer medications as usual practice.

Main outcomes measured:
- • Attitudes towards self-medication versus traditional care.
- • Satisfaction with self-medication.
- • Amounts of analgesia required by both groups.

Analysis:
- • The Likert summated rating scale with total scores was used to demonstrate how positive the respondents felt towards self-medication.
- • Triangulation was attempted using the data collected for analgesic requirements in the two groups. Unfortunately it was not possible and statistical evidence was tested by Mann Whitney U test alone.

Results:
Mothers in the self-medication group were very happy to take responsibility for their own medication scoring 83 per cent of the possible score on Likert scale. These mothers also needed less analgesia than mothers who had their medications administered by a midwife (p>0.05). Mothers from both groups were not aware of the effects and side effects of the medications they were taking.

Midwives were happy for mothers to have the choice to self-medicate but expressed concerns over safety issues.

Recommendations from this study:
Self-medication should be given serious consideration within a self care approach, as an expression of mothers' autonomy and choice.

Suggestions for further research:
Replication of this study could test the hypothesis that self-medication reduces the need for analgesia by measuring analgesia and analysing psychological effects of being in control.

Research into mothers' information and midwives' education about effects of medication, including effects on breastfeeding.

Additional relevant information:
One ward brought in a policy of self-medication in April 1996 and the other planned to follow soon afterwards. This will be audited in October 1996.

349. MIDWIVES' ASSESSMENT OF POSTNATAL UTERINE INVOLUTION: IMPLICATIONS FOR CLINICAL PRACTICE AND RESOURCE MANAGEMENT
January 1995–September 1997

Jo Alexander, Jo Garcia, Sally Marchant. **Contact:** Sally Marchant, Research Midwife, The National Perinatal Epidemiology Unit, Radcliffe Infirmary, Woodstock Road, Oxford, OX2 6HE. Tel: (01865) 224125/224875. Fax: (01865) 792270.

Funded as integral/additional part of a job by funding agency: South West Region Research and Development Committee.

Keywords: BLOOD LOSS ESTIMATION, CLINICAL JUDGEMENT, COMMUNITY CARE, CONCERNS (WOMEN'S), POSTNATAL CARE, POSTNATAL COMPLICATIONS, POSTNATAL EXAMINATION, POSTPARTUM HAEMORRHAGE (SECONDARY)

Aims of the study:
1. To identify women who present with bleeding problems from 24 hours after delivery until three months postnatally.
2. To describe the range of normal vaginal loss as reported by women during that time.
3. To determine antecedent factors which predispose to excessive bleeding in the postnatal period, including consideration of the predictive value of the routine assessment of uterine involution by midwives.

The research hypothesis is: 'Routine abdominal palpation of uterine fundal height in postnatal women, from 24 hours after delivery until the midwife discharges the mother from her care, fails to predict abnormal bleeding or uterine infection during the first three months postnatally'.

Ethics committee approval gained:
Yes

Research design:
Descriptive, qualitative, quantitative, survey, case control study.

Data Collection:
Techniques used:
Questionnaires, diaries, GP notification card survey (GPs have a pre-printed card to fill in for women who consult them with excessive or prolonged vaginal loss).

Case notes of women identified by selection criteria as having problems with excessive or prolonged vaginal loss. These notes were traced using the ICD codes, ward admission books, USS appointment records and GP notification cards.

Time data were collected:
Postnatal women between 24 hours and three months after delivery. GP prospective survey planned from July 1995 for 12 months. Retrospective case note review – two years, 1994 and 1995.

Testing of any tools used:
GP card piloted by six GPs. Women's survey piloted by 25 women in one district, using all tools. Case control piloted with 12 sets of notes.

Topics covered:
Range of normal vaginal loss in postnatal period.
Examples/incidence of uterine and vaginal blood loss problems (GPs and mothers).
Basic details of labour and delivery.
Review of midwifery observations of fundal height and vaginal loss.
Demographic details from participants.
Patterns of treatments and referrals.

In the case control:
- possible antecedent factors such as maternal age, parity, anaemia and physical health;
- birth weight, mode of delivery, details of third stage and infant feeding;
- comparison of postnatal midwifery observations.

Setting for data collection:
Hospital, urban and rural GP surgeries.

Details about sample studied:
Planned size of sample:
500 for women's survey.
At least 50 per cent of surgeries in each district.
Two controls per case.

Rationale for planned size:
Incidence of worst outcome (ERPC) 1 per cent. No estimates of less severe outcomes or treatments (USS, drug therapy).

Entry criteria:
Inclusion:
Women between 24 hours and three months post delivery.
GPs who have been consulted about excessive or prolonged bleeding 24 hours to three months post delivery.
Case notes of women who have had ERPC, USS or drug treatment for postnatal bleeding.

Exclusion:
Women excluded from survey on advice from staff.
Women who do not speak and write English.

Sample selection:
Data will be collected from the delivery register for all women delivering during the study period.

Interventions, Outcomes and Analysis:
Analysis:
SPSS for Windows. Descriptive statistics for women's survey. Statistical tests appropriate for mainly categorical data. Logistic regression for case control.

Marchant, S., Alexander, J. (1996). 'Midwives' assessment of postnatal uterine involution - is it of value?' Conference Proceedings, 24th Triennial Congress of the International Confederation of Midwives, pp 400–403. Oslo, International Confederation of Midwives.

Clinical studies: well and ill babies

229. BATHING NEWBORNS – IS HYPOTHERMIA INDUCED BY BATHING BABIES IMMEDIATELY AFTER DELIVERY?
May 1993–May 1996
C. K. Bates, J. Driver. **Contact:** K. Bates, Midwifery Sister, Queen Elizabeth Hospital, Gayton Road, King's Lynn, Norfolk PE32 2PJ. Tel: (01553) 613720.

6–12 hours/week of own time spent.

Keywords: BATHING, HYPOTHERMIA, INFANT NEWBORN, NEONATES

Aims of the study:
To establish whether babies become hypothermic if bathed immediately after delivery.

Ethics committee approval gained:
Yes

Research design:
Experimental, quantitative, randomized controlled trial.

Data Collection
Techniques used:
Records of observations.

Time data were collected:
At time of delivery and approximately 2 hours after delivery.

Testing of any tools used:
Piloted with 20 people.

Topics covered:
Room temperature
Rectal temperature of baby at birth
Rectal temperature of baby on admission to postnatal ward
Time of first feed
Apgar score
Type and time of delivery

Setting for data collection:
Hospital.

Details about sample studied:
Planned size of sample:
150

Rationale for planned size:
Represents one month's delivery numbers. One month chosen to prevent staff becoming de-motivated.

Entry criteria:
Inclusion:
> Gestational age 37+ weeks. Birthweight 2500–4500g. Apgar 7 or more at one minute.

Exclusion:
> Any baby with initial rectal temperature of <36°C.

Sample selection:
> Random

Actual sample size:
> 250

Interventions, Outcomes and Analysis:
Interventions used:
> Bathing the study group.

Main outcomes measured
> Rectal temperature change.

Analysis:
> Computer software

Results:
Statistical analysis showed no significant heat loss from babies who were bathed immediately after birth – hypothermia was not induced. Interestingly the results showed that the smaller and cooler the baby (within the inclusion criteria), the greater the increase in their body temperature if bathed.

406. SOME BELIEFS ABOUT COLOSTRUM AND REASONS FOR ITS OMISSION TO THE NEWBORN AMONG WOMEN FROM BANGLADESH

January 1990–September 1995

Catharine Littler. **Contact:** Catharine Littler, Research Midwife, Maternity Unit, Forest Healthcare Trust, Whipps Cross Hospital, Leytonstone, London E11 1NR. Tel: (0181) 539 5522 ext. 5833/5289. Fax: (0181) 558 8115.

Funded as integral additional part of a job by previous employer. Up to 2 hours/week of own time spent. Later written up in part fulfilment of a BHSc in Midwifery.

Keywords: ASIAN WOMEN, BREASTFEEDING, BREASTFEEDING (INFORMATION), BREASTFEEDING (STAFF KNOWLEDGE), BREASTFEEDING (SUPPLEMENTS), BREASTFEEDING BEHAVIOUR (MATERNAL), BREASTMILK, COLOSTRUM

Aims of the study:

The core research questions included:

- What do women from the Bangladeshi community and tradition believe about colostrum?
- Why does the practice of its omission exist?
- For how many days is colostrum omitted?
- Who or what influences these choices and beliefs?

Ethics committee approval gained:

Yes

Research design:

Descriptive, qualitative and quantitative, survey.

Data collection:
Techniques used:

Interviews and questionnaires

Time data were collected:

During a six month period in 1990–91

Testing of any tools used:

Ten mothers piloted the mothers' interview schedule, and five health professionals piloted their questionnaire. The questionnaire used a Likert scale.

Topics covered:

- Mothers: number of children and where they were born, knowledge and practice of infant feeding, influences on choice of feeding, beliefs about colostrum.
- Health professionals: length of time in post, perceptions of women's attitudes to infant feeding, whether and how they recommended early breastfeeding to mothers.

Setting for data collection:

Inner city hospital

Details about sample studied:
Planned size of sample:

60 newly delivered women from the Bangladeshi community. Staff on duty at the time of the study.

Rationale for planned size:

Convenience

Entry criteria:

Inclusions:

Healthy, recently delivered Bangladeshi women in the postnatal wards of the study hospital, after an uncomplicated vaginal delivery of a healthy baby, who consented to be interviewed.

Sample selection:
>   Convenience. The researcher visited the antenatal and postnatal wards with an interpreter on days when both were available, and approached women and staff about taking part in the study.

Actual sample size:
>   Women: 60
>   Staff: 23 (14 midwives, two student midwives, three nurses, two paediatricians – SHO and Registrar – and two obstetricians – SHO and Registrar).

Response rate:
>   100 per cent. All who were asked gave their consent.

Interventions, outcomes and analysis:
Analysis:
>   Content analysis, with SPSS for Likert scale; frequency values and percentages presented.

Results:
Ninety-eight per cent of the women fed their infants artificial milk in the first three days. Colostrum was hand expressed then discarded. The women decided to give or not to give the fluid they expressed on the grounds of its colour and density. Thin, watery fluid was omitted; thick, white fluid was given. Many of the health professionals thought the belief that colostrum is evil or harmful was the main reason why it was being omitted: the mothers said the watery fluid was 'too weak' for the infant, and that there was 'nothing in' the breast for the first three days. Women were more influenced in their feeding choices by other women than by their husbands, although there is evidence that this is changing.

Recommendations from this study:
*   Health education material should differentiate between colostrum and full breast milk to all women and in particular to women from the Bangladeshi community. Information should include the appearance and other attributes of colostrum as well as its role in the development of the immune system, and should be presented in the client's first language.
*   Bengali speaking maternity aides could influence the uptake of colostrum/breastfeeding, and managers should consider the importance of this role.
*   Transcultural midwifery education requires information such as that provided by this study, since there is evidence that feeding practices such as this exist in many parts of the world.

Suggestions for further research:
*   Do infants suffer from being given water/herbal fluids in the first three days?
*   How important is the principle of informed choice to the professional?

431. INFANT WEANING: LAY AND PROFESSIONAL ACCOUNTS OF THE WEANING PROCESS

September 1996–November 1998

J. M. Green; Gail Ewing, Research Associate. **Contact:** J. M. Green, Senior Lecturer, Midwifery Studies, University of Leeds, 22 Hyde Terrace, Leeds LS2 9LN. Tel: (0113) 233 6888. Fax: (0113) 244 9730.

Funded as part of a job by an award from Anglia and Oxford Regional Health Authority.

Keywords: CONFLICTING ADVICE (FEEDING), EXPECTATIONS (WOMEN'S), EXPERIENCE (WOMEN'S), INFANT FEEDING (DECISIONS), WEANING.

Aims of the study:

To investigate the process of normal weaning from both lay and professional perspectives, with particular reference to the common practice of early introduction of solid food to infants.

Ethics committee approval gained:

Yes

Research design:

Descriptive, qualitative and quantitative, comparative, grounded theory.

Data collection:
Techniques used:

First stage: focus groups with mothers and with Health Visitors. Main study: semistructured interviews, telephone interviews and questionnaires, with mothers.

Time data were collected:

Focus groups: mothers who have recently completed weaning their infants.
Main study: mothers from late pregnancy until their infants are six months old.

Testing of any tools used:

Questionnaires will be tested.

Topics covered:

Focus groups: the introduction of solid foods and discrepancies between official policy and practice.
Main study: all aspects of early infant care and behaviour.

Setting for data collection:

Focus groups in Health Centres. Main study in mothers' homes.

Details about sample studied:
Planned size of sample:
Four focus groups with eight mothers in each, and four with eight Health Visitors in each.
Main study: 40 mothers.

Rationale for planned size:
As large as practicable for qualitative data, and large enough to show statistically significant differences between groups if these exist.

Entry criteria:
Inclusions:
Any mother in the practices chosen for the study who is willing to take part and who speaks English.

Sample selection:
Convenience sample from local Health Centres. For the main study, the researchers aim to recruit 20 first time mothers and 20 with more than one child.

Actual sample size:
Not yet known.

Response rate:
• Not yet known.

Interventions, outcomes and analysis:
Main outcomes measured:
Main study: baby's age when solids first introduced.

Analysis:
Descriptive and simple comparative statistics for quantitative data. Atlas-ti software as an aid to grounded theory analysis.

Results:
Expected late 1998.

403. EVALUATION OF MATERNAL PHYSIOLOGIC RESPONSE TO MECHANICAL MILK EXPRESSION FOLLOWING PRETERM DELIVERY

March 1996–March 1998

Elizabeth Jones; S. A. Spencer, Consultant Neonatologist/Senior Lecturer. **Contact:** Elizabeth Jones, Breastfeeding Coordinator, Neonatal Unit, North Staffordshire Maternity Hospital, North Staffordshire NHS Trust, Newcastle Road, Stoke-on-Trent, Staffordshire ST4 6QG. Tel: (01782) 718440. Fax: (01782) 713401. Email: mea12@keele.ac.uk.
Funded by a charitable grant from Baby Lifeline. Up to 2 hours/week of own time spent.

Keywords: BREAST EXPRESSION, BREAST EXPRESSION (MECHANICAL), BREAST MASSAGE, BREASTFEEDING, BREASTFEEDING BEHAVIOUR (MATERNAL), BREASTMILK, PREMATURITY

Aims of the study:

1. To evaluate the effect of single and double (simultaneous) mechanical expression on milk volume and content following preterm delivery. Energy yield, acute and sustained response time will also be compared between the two groups.
2. To evaluate whether breast massage has a positive effect on milk removal response, milk yield and fat content.

Ethics committee approval gained:

Yes

Research design:

Experimental, quantitative, randomized controlled trial.

Data collection:
Techniques used:
Milk sampling, records of observations, medical records

Time data were collected:
4–10 days following preterm delivery (at less than 33 weeks gestation). Feeding data collected daily. Milk sampling after each expression.

Testing of any tools used:
Milk sampling (creamtocrit technique), validated by previous studies. All milk collections will be sampled to provide lipid analysis. This involves standard haemtocrit microtubes and a centrifuge. The percentage of cream is read from the capillary tube.
Egnell Ameda breast pumps are being used in the study because they create periodic and limited phases of negative pressure. It is thought that a cycle of pressure, rather than constant pressure maintenance, will avoid mammary tissue trauma.

Topics covered:
See under Main outcomes measured.

Setting for data collection:
Neonatal unit.

Details about sample studied:
Planned size of sample:
110 mothers, 55 in each arm of the trial.

Rationale for planned size:
Based on 80 per cent power at 5 per cent significance level.

Entry criteria:

Inclusions:

Mothers wishing to breastfeed infants born before 33 weeks gestation who consent to participate in the trial.

Exclusions:

Poor maternal health, retained products of conception.

Sample selection:

Random. The population has been stratified proportionate to gestational age. Sealed envelopes drawn randomly from each group will determine the trial population.

Actual sample size:

Not yet known

Response rate:

Not yet known

Interventions, outcomes and analysis:

Interventions used:

Mothers will be randomly allocated into two groups:
1.   Single pumping
2.   Double (simultaneous) pumping, for seven complete days.

All mothers in both groups will be asked to express milk eight times daily, at three hour intervals. The duration each expression will be dependent on breast emptying. All will use the same type of electric pump and lactation sets. All participants will be requested to alternate between massage or exclusive pump use on a daily basis. Massage involves gentle tactile stimulation of breast tissue involving a hand action that rolls the knuckles downwards over the breast, beginning at the ribs and working towards the areola. This technique does not involve manual expression of milk.

Main outcomes measured:

Milk volume, energy yield, total fat per volume, acute and sustained response time.

Analysis:

Standard deviation, correlation coefficients, quartile calculations, standard error of the difference in means, Chi-square.

Results:

September 1998.

413. HANDLING OF PREMATURE NEONATES: STUDY USING TIME-LAPSE VIDEO

November 1992–March 1993

Andrew Symon, Midwife, Steve Cunningham, Research Fellow. **Contact:** Andrew Symon, Staff Midwife, Maternity Unit, Perth Royal Infirmary, Perth PH1 1NX. Tel: (01738) 623311 ext. 3405. Fax: (01738) 628502.

Funded as integral part of a job by employer and by the Scottish Office (Chief Scientist's Office).

Keywords: MIDWIVES (NEONATAL), NEONATAL CARE, NEONATAL PROGRESS, PREMATURITY, RANDOMIZED CONTROLLED TRIAL

Aims of the study:
1. To assess whether the presence of continuous physiological trend data (heart rate, respiratory rate, $TcPO_2$, TcPCO levels) affected the incidence and duration of handling episodes in premature and very premature neonates.
2. To assess staff perceptions of such handling episodes.

Ethics committee approval gained:
Yes

Research design:
Experimental, quantitative, randomized controlled trial.

Data collection:
Techniques used:
Time lapse video, questionnaire.

Time data were collected:
At 6–30 hours of age, and at 48–72 hours of age.

Testing of any tools used:
Testing of the questionnaire was done with staff from the study unit.

Topics covered:
See Aims of the study

Setting for data collection:
Hospital neonatal unit.

Details about sample studied:
Planned size of sample:
20+

Rationale for planned size:
>Statistical analysis for matched pairs trial.

Entry criteria:
Inclusions:
>Babies of 32 weeks gestation or less, and babies who were ventilated or who were asphyxiated but not ventilated.

Sample selection:
>Those babies who were admitted to either of the two cot spaces covered by the video camera. Babies were matched retrospectively by gestational age.

Actual sample size:
>Twelve. The planned sample size was not reached because of 'blocking' of the two cot spaces concerned, i.e. a baby might remain in that cot space for some time after the video study had been competed.

Interventions, outcomes and analysis:
Interventions used:
>The researchers wanted to see whether having the screen data present affected the handling rate in either direction. Babies were randomized to having either the physiological trend data screen off (Group A, n=7) or having the screen on (Group B, n=5). There was no intention to treat babies in either group in a specific way.

Main outcomes measured:
>Incidence and duration of handling episodes, staff perceptions about these episodes.

Analysis:
>Data from analysis of time-lapse videos and staff questionnaires analysed using Microsoft Excel.

Results:
A large number of very brief handling episodes occurred for many of the babies. From this limited study no consistent correlation between handling rates and either gestational age or weight was found; nor did the presence of continuous trend monitoring appear to affect the incidence or duration of handling. Incidence and duration of handling episodes varied hugely, and it could not be concluded that physiological trend data was a factor. It had not been intended, nor was it possible, to identify exactly what a staff member was doing during a handling episode. Staff perceptions about handling varied enormously.

Recommendations from this study:
Education for staff is essential to minimize handling episodes.

Suggestions for further research:
Assessment of necessity of handling episodes.

Publications:
Symon, A., Cunningham, S. (1995) 'Handling premature neonates: a study using time-lapse video'. *Nursing Times* Vol. 91 No. 17, pp 35–37.

335. PROLONGING LIFE AND DECISION MAKING IN NEONATAL UNITS: THE THINKING AND PRACTICES OF DOCTORS AND NURSES

August 1994–June 1996
Hazel McHaffie, Peter Fowlie. **Contact:** Hazel E. McHaffie, Research Fellow, Institute of Medical Ethics, University of Edinburgh, Department of Medicine, Royal Infirmary, Lauriston Place, Edinburgh, EH3 9YW. Tel: (0131) 536 1827.

Funded as integral/additional part of a job by funding agency: Chief Scientist Office, Scottish Office Home and Health Department, St Andrew's House, Edinburgh, EH1 3DE.

Keywords: CONFLICT, DECISION MAKING, ETHICS, LAW, NEONATES

Aims of the study:
To explore thinking and practices amongst doctors and nurses in relation to decision making in Neonatal Intensive Care Units in cases where withdrawal or withholding of treatment are possible options. To do this with special reference to ethical reasoning, perceived dilemmas, sources of conflict and productive working practices.

Ethics committee approval gained:
Yes

Research design:
Descriptive, qualitative, survey.

>**Data Collection:**
>>**Techniques used:**
>>>Interviews, observation.

>>**Time data were collected:**
>>>October 1994–September 1995.

>>**Testing of any tools used:**
>>>Interview schedules were tested with professionals from neonatal units other than those selected for the main study.

Topics covered:
>Perceptions of the law
>Procedures for decision making
>Dilemmas encountered
>Sources of conflict and tension
>Roles and responsibilities
>Factors which influence behaviour and thinking re ethical issues
>Support systems
>Education

Setting for data collection:
>Six neonatal units – four University based Hospitals and two District General Hospitals.

Details about sample studied:
Planned size of sample:
>Minimum 50 doctors, 50 nurses.

Rationale for planned size:
>Sufficient to saturate categories for analysis.

Entry criteria:
Inclusion:
>Stratified sample of trained staff working in neonatal units. All consultants given the opportunity to participate.

Exclusion:
>Students

Sample selection:
>Convenience

Actual sample size:
>57 doctors, 119 nurses/midwives.

Response rate:
>Impossible to quantify.

Interventions, Outcomes and Analysis:
Analysis:
>Microsoft Excel and SPSS pc.

Results:
1. Clinicians take these important decisions very seriously.
2. Knowledge of the law is hazy but some situations, such as the use of drugs and the withdrawal of nourishment, are grey areas which cause considerable problems.
3. Staff are influenced by a range of personal as well as professional factors, with experience in caring for very sick, impaired and premature infants affecting them profoundly.

4. Procedures and practices differ both between Units and between consultants. Junior staff can be caught in untenable positions where consultants disagree.
5. The majority of staff believe that cases should be considered on their own merits closely involving the family in the decision making process. Judgements about quality of life are often inevitable but opinions vary considerably about where lines should be drawn relating to burdens and benefits.
6. The timing of events is a major cause of conflict with interpersonal conflict adding to the tension created. The management of certain infants such as the severely birth asphyxiated whose prognosis is poor but who do not require intensive aggressive therapy, is a particularly difficult area of practice producing stress and conflict.

Recommendations from this study:
In order for NICU teams to operate most effectively:
• both doctors and nurses need to be critically aware of their own values and opinions about life and death issues as well as those of their colleagues and the parents
• staff should be encouraged actively to participate in discussion around treatment decisions as well as in the management of babies for whom treatment might not be the best option
• as team leaders, consultants should be involved throughout, consistent in their practices, and sensitive to the needs and views of colleagues and parents
• resources should be made available to prepare staff for and support them in these difficult situations. Adequate staffing levels, ongoing education, and the provision of a recognised support system are some of the ways identified which might help to reduce stress and tension.

Suggestions for further research:
Being involved in decisions relating to withdrawal or withholding of treatment has been seen to be fraught with tension and potential conflict for staff. But for parents it would seem to be a profoundly stressful experience. Only they can identify their needs and wishes. A complementary study is needed to explore their perspective in order to assess the adequacy of current practices, bereavement care and follow up services. A study to address these issues commenced in the Institute of Medical Ethics in July 1996.

McHaffie, H.E., Fowlie, P.W. (1996) *Life, Death and Decisions: Doctors and Nurses Reflect on Neonatal Practice.* Hale: Hochland and Hochland Ltd
McHaffie, H.E., Fowlie, P.W. (1996) *Life, Death and Decisions: Doctors and Nurses Reflect on Neonatal Practice. An Executive Summary.* Hale: Hochland and Hochland Ltd

Clinical studies: women's views

400. WOMEN'S EXPERIENCE OF WATERBIRTH
October 1993–September 1994
Helen Richmond. **Contact:** Helen Richmond, via MIRIAD office.

Funded as part of a course by The Smith and Nephew Foundation, and by the Hospital Saving Association Charitable Trust. 6–12 hours per week of own time spent.

Keywords: EXPECTATIONS (WOMEN'S), EXPERIENCE (WOMEN'S), OUTCOMES (NEONATAL), PAIN RELIEF (LABOUR), PERCEPTIONS OF CHILDBIRTH (WOMEN'S), PERCEPTIONS OF PAIN (WOMEN'S), WATER BIRTH, WOMEN'S VIEWS

Aims of the study:
To address two questions:
1. What are the experiences of women who have had a waterbirth?
2. Do all women perceive waterbirth as therapeutic?

Ethics committee approval gained:
Yes

Research design:
Descriptive, qualitative and quantitative, survey.

Data collection:
Techniques used:
Postal questionnaire.

Time data were collected:
1–3 years after the waterbirth.

Testing of any tools used:
Used material from taped interviews with nine women to produce pilot questionnaire. Questionnaire piloted with four mothers representing different social classes and ethnic groups, a GP and an NCT teacher, all from one geographical area. Questionnaire repiloted with two mothers from another area and a midwife colleague, before being sent out. Social class coded using Standard Occupational Classification (OPCS, 1991).

Topics covered:
1. Mothers' age, social class and qualifications.
2. Where mothers first heard about waterbirth, why they chose waterbirth, antenatal preparation for waterbirth.
3. Mothers' feelings on first entering the pool, length of time spent in the pool, pain relief used when in the water.
4. What mothers particularly liked/disliked about waterbirth, how pleasurable/painful was the experience, did the waterbirth meet their expectations.
5. Behaviour differences between babies born in and out of water.
6. Would mothers have another waterbirth.
7. General comments.

Setting for data collection:
> Postal survey.

Details about sample studied:
Planned size of sample:
> 240 women.

Rationale for planned size:
> The total number of women who had experienced waterbirth in one county in South East England from 1991 to 1993 was 482. The study aimed for a 50 per cent sample.

Entry criteria:
Inclusions:
> Birth in water.

Exclusions:
> Women whose babies had Apgar scores below 7 at one minute (41) and women whose babies suffered a neonatal death (2) were excluded for ethical reasons.

Sample selection:
> After exclusions, one in two deliveries in water, in the order of the births, in the time and area studied.

Actual sample size:
> 240 questionnaires sent out.

Response rate:
> 189 responses received (79 per cent).

Interventions, outcomes and analysis:
Analysis:
> Data loaded onto EXCEL spreadsheet then downloaded onto floppy disc in Lotus 1,2,3 format in order to be assessed by the Standard Package for the Social Services (SPSS). Statistical tests performed by SPSS included Spearman's Rho and chi-squared test.

Results:
1. The respondents were mainly well educated and middle class.
2. 145 (78 per cent) of the mothers wanted waterbirth for pain relief and 73 per cent for a 'natural', gentle birth for their baby. A few were prepared antenatally for waterbirth.
3. Mothers repeatedly used the words relaxation, relief, pain relief and warmth to describe their feelings on entering the pool. Many of the mothers used Entonox when in the water.

4. Mothers felt more 'in control' of themselves and their environment when in the water and this was important to them. They particularly liked the relaxing quality of the water, the physical support it gave them, and being able to hold their babies immediately after birth. A small minority of women did not enjoy waterbirth, finding the environment too hot and fearing the baby might drown. 18 per cent found waterbirth less painful than expected and 72 per cent as painful as expected. 49 per cent found waterbirth better than expected and 50 per cent as expected.

5. There were doubts about the reliability of the measurement used for comparing the behaviour of babies born in and out of water. No statistically significant differences were found. Those who had any worries about their waterborn babies thought they were due to the waterbirth or the midwife.

6. 160 mothers (85 per cent) thought waterbirth was therapeutic and 81 per cent were strongly in favour of having another labour and birth in water.

7. Fifteen mothers (8 per cent) criticised facilities and fourteen mothers (7 per cent) criticised midwife training for waterbirth.

Recommendations from this study:

It was important for women in this study to feel 'in control' and to be able to hold their baby immediately after the birth. Midwives could meet these needs for women in or out of water. Where a waterbirth service is offered, midwives need supervisory and managerial support as well as up to date knowledge and skills, and they should discuss the available facts about waterbirth with women before delivery in water takes place. Antenatal preparation for waterbirth may reduce the use of Entonox in the pool, and should emphasise that if deviations from normal occur, the mother will be asked to get out of the water. Units offering waterbirth should share their expertise.

Suggestions for further research:

This study was biased towards mothers who had a good experience of waterbirth. Even so, a few did not have good experiences. There is an urgent need to audit and evaluate outcomes of waterbirth on a national scale, and to follow up all babies born in water, so that the benefits and hazards of this practice can be fully evaluated.

Related study:

239. PRELIMINARY EVALUATION OF HYDROTHERAPY IN LABOUR, USING HARD INDICATORS
The abstract appears on p.34 under *Clinical studies: birth and after.*

419. HOME BIRTH
June 1993–September 1996

Geoffrey Chamberlain, Professor of Obstetrics and Gynaecology, Ann Wraight, Research Midwife, Patricia Crowley, Obstetrician. **Contact:** Ann Wraight, via MIRIAD office.

Funded by a contract from the National Birthday Trust Fund of the Royal College of Obstetricians and Gynaecologists.

Keywords: CHILDBIRTH (CONTROL OF), EXPERIENCE (MIDWIVES'), EXPERIENCE (WOMEN'S), HOME BIRTHS, INFORMED CHOICE, OUTCOMES (MATERNAL), OUTCOMES (NEONATAL), PLACE OF BIRTH

Aims of the study:

1. To obtain a contemporary account of home births in the UK in 1994 from the professionals and the women having babies in that year.
2. To assess the outcome of those who planned to give birth at home compared with those who planned to give birth in hospital. This was to include physical measures, opinions and views of the women and the professionals.

Ethics committee approval gained:

Yes

Research design:

Descriptive, qualitative and quantitative, survey.

Data collection:
Techniques used:

Two postal questionnaire surveys.

Time data were collected:

1. Within 48 hours of giving birth.
2. 6–8 weeks postnatal (20 per cent random sample).

Testing of any tools used:

1. Questionnaires piloted by 8 postnatal mothers in a London teaching hospital.
2. Questionnaires tested by 20 mothers and midwives in two hospitals and community areas (one city, one rural).

Topics covered:

Experience, outcome and satisfaction, for births at home and in hospital.

Setting for data collection:

Hospitals and women's homes in urban and rural areas.

Details about sample studied:
Planned size of sample:

All births planned, at 37 weeks gestation, to take place at home in 1994 in UK: 1.5–2 per cent of total births that year.

Rationale for planned size:

To provide a picture of women's views nationally (last survey 1979).

To exclude from the planned home birth group those whose pregnancies did not reach term and those whose booking was changed before term.

Entry criteria:

Inclusions:

All women who consented at 37 weeks gestation having been booked for home birth, irrespective of where the birth took place. As controls, women with similar backgrounds, who consented at 37 weeks having been booked for hospital birth.

Sample selection:

No sampling for main survey.
Random sample for follow up survey (20 per cent).

Actual sample size:

6004 planned home births, 4621 planned hospital births.
Follow up questionnaire sent to a random 20 per cent.

Response rate:

Main survey: 5971 from planned home birth group (98 per cent), 4531 from planned hospital birth group (98 per cent).
Follow up: 855 responses from planned home birth group, 645 responses from planned hospital birth group.

Interventions, outcomes and analysis:

Analysis:

The SPSS system was used to access and analyse the data. Simple frequency and cross tabulations were done on the total populations and on subsets. Chi-squared tests were used to investigate the association between categorical variables such as place of birth and social class.

Results:

In preparation.

Additional relevant information:

The study includes a small section on unplanned home births, n=1600.

395. THE MEANING AND IMPORTANCE OF CHILDBIRTH FOR PRIMIPAROUS WOMEN

September 1994–April 1995

Kate Dixon. **Contact:** Kate Dixon, via MIRIAD office.

Formed part of BSc (Midwifery) course. More than 20 hours/week spent on the research. No additional funding was obtained.

Keywords: EXPERIENCE (WOMEN'S), GROUNDED THEORY, MATERNITY CARE EXPERIENCE, PERCEPTIONS OF CHILDBIRTH (WOMEN'S), PERCEPTIONS OF MOTHERHOOD (WOMEN'S), PRIMIPARAE

Aims of the study:
To explore the meaning and importance of childbirth for primiparous women.

Ethics committee approval gained:
Yes

Research design:
Descriptive, qualitative.

Data collection:
Techniques used:
Open-ended interviews.

Time data were collected:
Approximately 6 months postnatally.

Testing of any tools used:
An interview topic guide was constructed, but not rigidly adhered to.

Topics covered:
The social, spiritual, psychological, emotional, mental and physical importance and meaning of childbirth.

Setting for data collection:
Women's homes, in an urban setting in the South of England.

Details about sample studied:
Planned size of sample:
6–12

Rationale for planned size:
Small, so that the information from each participant could be analysed in depth.

Entry criteria:
Inclusions:
Women who had their first baby in the study unit during May-June 1994, whose delivery details in the labour ward register included their full address, and who returned a signed consent form.

Sample selection:
Purposive. Consent forms were sent out to all the twenty women who met the study criteria. Seven were returned and these women were interviewed.

Actual sample size:
Seven

Response rate:
N/A

Interventions, outcomes and analysis:
Analysis:
Used an adaptation of grounded theory, with some similarities to symbolic interactionist analysis. Interviews transcribed and original codes and categories formed, then five major categories that were relevant to all respondents, including a core category. Constant comparison followed until saturation; storyline formulated, demonstrating typicality. Ideas emerged.

Results:
The five major categories were: trusting the professional (core category), being in limbo, the intensity of pain, reality shock, and achieving something special.

The women interviewed all trusted the professionals involved, perceiving them as experts doing the best to care for both mother and baby. The women felt vulnerable, 'in limbo' throughout their labour and birth. They were shocked at the intensity of labour pain, childbirth and suturing, the enormity of childbirth and the implications of caring for a fully dependent baby. Not only did it take a long time for the reality of the birth to sink in, it also took them many months to adapt to family life. These women perceived birth as an achievement. Regardless of interventions or mode of delivery, they were proud at having brought a life into the world.

Recommendations from this study:
Women in the study spoke with feeling about their needs for improved antenatal education, a flexible approach to communication, more support during suturing, the presence of their families, individual breastfeeding advice and increased awareness of individual differences. Midwives may find that other women share these needs.

Suggestions for further research:
An antenatal study of what women pregnant for the first time think childbirth will mean for them could be followed up postnatally to find out how the same women interpret their actual experience.

All the women interviewed appreciated the opportunity to talk. It could be that increased debriefing facilities have a value in the detection and possibly the prevention of postnatal depression.

399. CAN WOMEN HAVE IT ALL? – MOTHERHOOD AND A CAREER

January 1994–October 1994
Lynn Smith. **Contact:** Lynn Smith, Senior Midwife Teacher, European Institute of Health and Medical Sciences, Silverlands Campus, Holloway Hill, Lyne, Chertsey, Surrey KT16 0AE. Tel: (01932) 874161. Fax: (01932) 875447.

Formed part of a course. Employer paid course fees and gave 43 study days per year. 6–12 hours per week of own time spent.

Keywords: ADAPTATION TO MOTHERHOOD, CAREER PATHS, CHILDBIRTH (SOCIAL FACTORS), EMPLOYMENT, WOMEN'S VIEWS

Aims of the study:
To ascertain the views and experiences of a selected group of first time mothers who were also working in professional employment about whether motherhood and a career could coexist.

Ethics committee approval gained:
No. The Clinical Director of Obstetrics and Gynaecology gave permission to access records to identify the women in the study group. The women chose to participate after explanation of their proposed role in the study.

Research design:
Descriptive, qualitative, ethnography.

Data collection:
Techniques used:
Interviews, taped and transcribed verbatim. Interview notes.

Time data were collected:
The women in the study group were taking maternity leave from work and were 8–12 weeks postnatal.

Testing of any tools used:
None

Topics covered:
Interview schedule focused on the following topics:
- Views on their own mothering and why they chose to be mothers
- Views on their work and the combining of this with the mother role
- Division of labour within the home
- Reactions of their mothers to the combining of work and mothering

Setting for data collection:
Women's homes.

Details about sample studied:
Planned size of sample:
Ten primiparous women.

Rationale for planned size:
Reasonable number from whom to obtain and analyse interview data in the time available.

Entry criteria:
Inclusions:
Primiparous women working in 'male dominated' professions (medicine, law, accountancy), intending to return to work after maternity leave.

Sample selection:
Convenience. Sixteen women who met the inclusion criteria were identified from antenatal booking database records and invited to participate. Eight agreed.

Actual sample size:
Five women.

Interventions, outcomes and analysis:
Analysis:
Intensive scrutiny of the transcripts of interviews and the interview notes. Several categories emerged from the data which were compared and contrasted with the literature reviewed.

Results:
Four major themes emerged:
- Life chances have opened up for these women enabling them to participate in both public and private spheres.
- Although becoming a mother was a carefully planned event and warmly welcomed, the women in the study group knew that the mother role alone was insufficient for them.
- All the women were married, and their husbands appeared from the data not to be threatened either by taking on a mothering role or by being less successful in career terms than their wives.
- There is blurring of gender roles within these couples and as a result, motherhood and a career were not seen as mutually exclusive.

Suggestions for further research:
It would be interesting to follow up the study group to ascertain how their lived reality of returning to work compared with their expectations and plans at the time of the study.

424. A MODIFIED REPLICATION OF THE OPCS SURVEY OF WOMEN'S EXPERIENCE OF CHILDBIRTH USING A POSTNATAL QUESTIONNAIRE

November 1994–May 1995

Valerie Rowett. **Contact:** Valerie Rowett, Midwifery Sister, Manygates Maternity Unit, Pinderfields General Hospital, Aberford Road, Wakefield, West Yorks WF1 4DG. Tel: (01924) 814935.

Formed part of a course. Employer funded half course fees and stationery. 12–20 hours/week of own time spent.

Keywords: ANTENATAL CARE, CHANGING CHILDBIRTH, EXPERIENCE (WOMEN'S), LABOUR (CARE), LABOUR (SATISFACTION), POSTNATAL CARE, WOMEN'S VIEWS

Aims of the study:
- To survey women's views of the care they received from the maternity unit studied.
- To ascertain whether the local maternity service was meeting the main objective of 'Changing Childbirth' (1993) of a 'woman centred' approach to care, based on women's individual needs.
- To provide information for a local policy review of maternity services.

Ethics committee approval gained:
Yes

Research design:
Descriptive, qualitative and quantitative, survey.

Data collection:
Techniques used:
Questionnaire

Time data were collected:
Questionnaires distributed on transfer home from the postnatal ward and returned on discharge from the community midwife.

Testing of any tools used:
A modified version of a previously tried and tested questionnaire was used (Mason, 1989).

Topics covered:
Aspects of antenatal care, labour and delivery; postnatal stay in hospital, community care; level of satisfaction with care, women's views about the care they received.

Setting for data collection:
Women's homes

Details about sample studied:
Planned size of sample:
Approximately 200

Rationale for planned size:
One month's deliveries in the study unit.

Entry criteria:
Inclusions:
Women who gave birth in the unit during November 1994.

Exclusions:
Women who had a stillbirth, a neonatal death or an ill baby, women who gave birth outside the Unit (home births or BBAs), women who lived out of the area, women who could not read and write in English, women who declined participation.

Sample selection:
Convenience

Actual sample size:
160 deliveries during November 1994. Following exclusions, 109 questionnaires were sent out.

Response rate:
65 questionnaires returned (60 per cent).

Interventions, outcomes and analysis:
Analysis:
Numerical data from returned questionnaires were analysed using computer programme Paradox. A percentage analysis of edited data was carried out; significant results were then expanded upon.

Results:
Overall, satisfaction levels were high, with many positive answers about the current service as a whole. Important common themes were quality of information, friendliness and involvement of partner. There was a variety of views about wanting to get to know caregivers antenatally. Women reported high levels of satisfaction about labour and delivery without necessarily knowing their care-giver. There was least satisfaction with postnatal care in hospital. Views about this were sometimes contradictory and were concerned with issues such as 'poor quality of meals' and 'staff being too busy' as well as direct midwifery care. Community care was often described as excellent. There is evidence to suggest a woman centred approach to care in the unit. However, it appeared that at the same time the use of obstetric technology such as electronic fetal monitoring was standard practice.

Recommendations from this study:
Women's views should to be continually assessed to ensure woman centred care.

Suggestions for further research:
Observational study of health professionals to determine to what extent women are offered informed choices. Comparison study of caregivers at the beginning and end of pregnancy, to assess continuity of carers. Studies to compare use of obstetric technology under consultant care and midwife care.

Related study:
384. GETTING CONSUMERS' VIEWS OF MATERNITY SERVICES
The abstract appears on p.117 under *Management studies*.

428. EXPLORING DIFFERENCES IN WOMEN'S EXPERIENCES OF PREGNANCY AND EARLY MOTHERHOOD

June 1995–November 1996

J. M. Green; Kostas Kafetsios, Research Assistant. **Contact:** J. M. Green, Senior Lecturer, Midwifery Studies, University of Leeds, 22 Hyde Terrace, Leeds LS2 9LN. Tel: (0113) 233 6888. Fax: (0113) 244 9730.

Funded as part of a job by an award from the Health Promotion Research Trust, Cambridge.

Keywords: ADAPTATION TO MOTHERHOOD, BREASTFEEDING (DURATION), BREASTFEEDING (INTENTION), EDINBURGH POSTNATAL DEPRESSION SCALE, EXPECTATIONS (WOMEN'S), MATERNAL CHARACTERISTICS, PERCEPTIONS OF MOTHERHOOD (WOMEN'S), WOMEN'S VIEWS

Aims of the study:

The grant was for secondary analysis of a large data set from a longitudinal study which followed women from pre-booking until six weeks after delivery. The aim was to use multivariate statistical techniques to discover more about determinants of different women's experiences.

Ethics committee approval gained:

Not required for secondary analysis.

Research design:

Secondary analysis, multivariate statistical analysis.

Data collection:

None was collected in this part of the study. The following section refers to the earlier part of the study, PSYCHOLOGICAL AND SOCIAL ASPECTS OF SCREENING DURING ROUTINE ANTENATAL CARE, reported in the 1994 edition of MIRIAD (study 77).

Techniques used:

Questionnaires

Time data were collected:

At 16 weeks of pregnancy (or before antenatal booking if this was later), at 22 and 35 weeks of pregnancy and at 6 weeks after the birth.

Testing of any tools used:

All questionnaires were piloted.

Topics covered:

Maternity care – feelings, attitudes, experiences, relationships. Demographic details.

Setting for data collection:
Postal questionnaire.

Details about sample studied:
Planned size of sample:
1800 women

Rationale for planned size:
200 from each of nine districts

Entry criteria:
Inclusions:
All women booked for antenatal care at the study units during the study period who gave their consent.

Sample selection:
Unselected group of women at hospitals with different screening policies.

Actual sample size:
2325 (a linked study recruited a further 500 women from the Midlands).

Response rate:
Highly variable between hospitals.

Interventions, outcomes and analysis:
Main outcomes measured:
Emotional wellbeing postnatally, breastfeeding rates.

Analysis:
Multiple regression, factorial analysis of variance, log linear modelling.

Results:
In preparation.

Green, J.M., Kafetsios, K. 'Positive experiences of early motherhood: predictive variables from a longitudinal study'. *Journal of Reproductive and Infant Psychology* (in press).

Clinical studies:
midwives and midwifery

260. FACILITATING INFORMED CHOICE IN CHILDBIRTH: A STUDY OF MIDWIVES AND THEIR CLIENTS
September 1993–September 1997
Valerie A. Levy. **Contact:** Valerie Levy, Senior Lecturer, The Chinese University of Hong Kong, Department of Nursing, Shatin, Hong Kong.

Formed part of a course. Funded as integral/additional part of a job by employer and funding agency: Smith and Nephew Foundation. 6–12 hours/week of own time spent.

Keywords: DECISION MAKING, INFORMATION GIVING, INFORMED CHOICE, PREGNANCY, GROUNDED THEORY

Aims of the study:
To investigate issues relating to informed decision making by women during pregnancy. Processes to be explored include:
a) midwives facilitating decision making;
b) women engaging in the processes of facilitation and decision making.

Ethics committee approval gained:
Yes

Research design:
Descriptive, qualitative, ethnography, grounded theory.

Data Collection:
Techniques used:
Records of observations, interviews.

Time data were collected:
Booking clinics and later in pregnancy.

Setting for data collection:
Hospital, community.

Details about sample studied:
Planned size of sample:
Not planned as using grounded theory.

Rationale for planned size:
Theoretical sampling.

Sample selection:
In line with emerging themes.

Actual sample size:
Recruitment ongoing.

Interventions, Outcomes and Analysis:
  Analysis:
    Constant comparative analysis.

Results:
Ongoing.

411. MIDWIVES WITHOUT CHILDREN: A PHENOMENO-LOGICAL STUDY OF RELATIONSHIPS
November 1994–August 1995
Christine Bewley. **Contact:** Mrs. Chris Bewley, Senior Lecturer, Middlesex University, Faculty of Health Studies, 10 Highgate Hill, London N19 5ND. Tel: (0171) 288 5932. Fax: (0171) 288 5103.

Formed part of a course. Course funded by employer (time and £400 pa) and by the King's Fund (£200 pa). 2–6 hours/week of own time spent.

Keywords: COMMUNICATION SKILLS, EXPERIENCE (MIDWIVES'), INTRAPROFESSIONAL SUPPORT, MIDWIFE-MOTHER RELATIONSHIP, PERCEPTIONS OF CHILDBIRTH (WOMEN'S), PERCEPTIONS OF MOTHERHOOD (WOMEN'S), PERCEPTIONS OF PARENTHOOD (MIDWIVES'), THERAPEUTIC RELATIONSHIP

Aims of the study:
To gain insight into the attitudes and approaches to childbearing women of midwives who themselves do not have children.

Ethics committee approval gained:
Yes

Research design:
Descriptive, qualitative, phenomenology.

  Data collection:
    Techniques used:
      Interviews, field notes and the researcher's reflective diary.

    Time data were collected:
      January 1995.

    Testing of any tools used:
      Research question piloted with colleagues. All analysed results discussed with participants.

    Topics covered:
      Participants' responses to the question 'Do you have children?'

Setting for data collection:
Hospital

Details about sample studied:
Planned size of sample:
Six midwives.

Rationale for planned size:
Manageable for one researcher.

Entry criteria:
Inclusions:
Midwives without children for any reason, as at 1 December 1994.

Exclusions:
Midwives with living children.

Sample selection:
Purposive.

Actual sample size:
Six midwives.

Response rate:
N/A

Interventions, outcomes and analysis:
Analysis:
Analysis of interview transcripts and extraction of formulated meanings, which formed sub-themes and themes.

Results:
The findings suggested that midwives were frequently asked by clients if they had children. Although the question constituted part of a social interaction, some perceived it as a personal question containing an element of threat. Respondents sought to maintain professional credibility and assure women of compassionate care despite lack of a shared experience. Most felt that professional expertise was more important than the experience of pregnancy. Some felt the need to justify their childlessness emphasising that they wanted children in the future. Some used joking responses to the question 'have you got children?', which had the effect of preventing further conversation on the subject. This technique was used by one midwife who knew she could not have children, with the specific intent of protecting herself from further questioning.

Recommendations from this study:
Childless midwives and student midwives need support in situations which may threaten their professional credibility or cause them to feel alienated.

422. AN EXPLORATION OF THE SUPPORT OFFERED TO WOMEN IN LABOUR FROM THE MIDWIFE'S PERSPECTIVE
November 1993–November 1994

Margaret Lynch. **Contact:** Margaret Lynch, Midwife Teacher, Manchester College of Midwifery and Nursing, Gateway House, Piccadilly South, Manchester M60 7LP. Tel: (0161) 237 2260. Fax: (0161) 237 2913.

Funded by employer as part of an MSc in Practitioner Research. 6–12 hours/week of own time spent.

Keywords: EMOTIONAL LABOUR, EXPERIENCE (MIDWIVES'), LABOUR, MIDWIFE-MOTHER RELATIONSHIP, MIDWIFERY SUPPORT, SOCIAL SUPPORT

Aims of the study:
To explore the issue of support offered to women in labour from the perspective of the midwives giving that support. To explore what forms that support takes, what influences the amount and type of support given, and the relationship between the supporters as seen by the midwives involved in the study.

Ethics committee approval gained:
No. Individual staff consented, and consent from manager to interview staff was obtained. Women/clients/partners/families were not involved.

Research design:
Descriptive, qualitative, survey.

> **Data collection:**
> > **Techniques used:**
> > Semistructured interviews based on scenarios and events in different labour contexts.
>
> > **Time data were collected:**
> > N/A
>
> > **Testing of any tools used:**
> > Interview schedule tested with four midwives.
>
> > **Topics covered:**
> > Support offered by midwives to women in labour. What forms did support take. What influences the amount and type of support offered. Relationship between the supporting midwife and other supporters.
>
> > **Setting for data collection:**
> > An urban hospital.

Details about sample studied:
Planned size of sample:
20 midwives

Rationale for planned size:
Manageable, and sufficient for an exploratory study.

Entry criteria:
Inclusions:
Midwives working in the study hospital.

Sample selection:
The hospital's personnel department supplied a random list of midwives stratified to represent day and night staff on grades E, F and G.

Actual sample size:
20

Response rate:
15 (75 per cent)

Interventions, outcomes and analysis:
Analysis:
All interviews were fully transcribed and analysed. Content analysis based on Burnard's (1991) thematic content model.

Results:
Midwives reported offering the following forms of support: information giving, physical support in the form of touch (back rubbing and hand holding), and advocacy (by empowering women to speak for themselves rather than speaking for them). Emotional support, described by other authors (see Additional relevant information) as 'emotional labour', was a major category in relation to all the scenarios.

The amount and type of support offered appeared to be influenced by the midwife's impression or stereotype of the labouring woman (for example, whether she was a pregnant teenager, 'high risk', a member of an ethnic minority or wished to have a low technology active labour). Other influences included the presence or absence of a partner or other support person, and workload on the unit. A senior and junior partnership model emerged as the way in which midwives view their relationship with other supporters, the midwife seeing herself as senior partner.

Recommendations from this study:
The concept of 'emotional labour' highlights important aspects of the role of the midwife which should be encouraged and valued.

Suggestions for further research:
Further work needs to be done on 'emotional labour', and on if and how aptitude for it can be identified in potential recruits to midwifery.

Additional relevant information:
The researcher cites the following work by others around the concept of emotional labour:

Hodnett, E., Osborne E. (1989) 'A randomized trial on the effects of monitrice support during labour.' *Birth*, 16, pp.177–78.

James, N. (1987) 'Emotional labour: skill and work in the social regulation of feelings.' *Sociological Review* 37(1) pp.15–42.

Klaus, M., Kennell, J., Robertson S., Sosa R. (1986) 'Effects of social support during parturition on maternal infant morbidity.' *British Medical Journal* Vol. 293 pp.585–87.

420. ACTIVITIES, RESPONSIBILITIES AND INDEPENDENCE OF MIDWIVES WITHIN THE EUROPEAN UNION
December 1989–May 1996

Ruth Ashton OBE, Honorary Secretary/Treasurer of the European Midwives Liaison Committee (EMLC) (retired), Pamela Jennings, Head of Midwifery (retired), Angela Smith, Midwife Teacher (retired), Keith Jacka, Statistician (retired). **Contact:** Mrs. Marianne Mead, Administrator, EMLC, 7 Dalestones, West Hunsbury, Northampton NN4 9UU. Tel: (01604) 702121. Email: 106072.156@compuserve.com

Ruth Ashton took overall responsibility for this study in her own time as part of her role as Honorary Secretary/Treasurer of the EMLC. Midwifery associations of eight EC countries provided funds or funded their own postage for the study. Additional funds were obtained from The Edwina Mountbatten Trust, The European Union Small Grants, and The Royal National Pension fund for Nurses.

Keywords: ACCOUNTABILITY, DECISION MAKING, EXPERIENCE (MIDWIVES'), INTERNATIONAL MIDWIFERY, LEARNING ENVIRONMENT, MIDWIFERY PRACTICE

Aims of the study:
The aim of the project was:
- to make a quantitative assessment of the activities, responsibilities and independence of midwives within the European Union (EU);
- to compare the above with the competencies which are required by the Midwives' directives for the training of midwives (Directive 80/155/EEC, Article 4: see under Additional relevant information);
- to assess the extent to which the competencies were used by practising midwives to quantify the responsibility taken and the independence of midwives within the member states.

Ethics committee approval gained:
No

Research design:
Descriptive, quantitative, survey.

Data collection:
Techniques used:
Questionnaires to the following in each EC member state:
1. The competent authority (midwives registering body);
2. Chief midwives/Heads of midwifery services;
3. Midwives in practice.

Time data were collected:
1. 1989;
2.& 3. 1992–3

Testing of any tools used:
Questionnaires were based on the list of activities which EU member states must ensure midwives are at least entitled to take up and pursue (Directive 80/155/EEC Article 4). Questionnaires for the chief midwives and midwives in practice were piloted in Denmark and the UK.

Topics covered:
1. The competent authorities were asked if midwives in their state were permitted to undertake each activity.
2. Chief midwives were asked if midwives in the unit they managed undertook the full range of activities contained in the Directive.
3. Midwives in practice were asked if they undertook the activities contained in the list.

Setting for data collection:
Postal survey throughout Europe.

Details about sample studied:
Planned size of sample:
A percentage of the midwives in each EC country, with a maximum of 1000 from each country. The exceptions were Luxembourg, where all 62 midwives received a questionnaire, and Germany, where additional questionnaires were circulated to accommodate the additional number of midwives following reunification.

Rationale for planned size:
Statistical advice that results would be generalisable given a 50 per cent response rate.

Entry criteria:
Inclusions:
1. The competent authority in each EC member state;
2. Chief midwives in these countries;
3. Midwives registered with the competent authority of an EC member state.

Sample selection:
1. All the competent authorities;
2. Each country's competent authority was asked to send a questionnaire to each chief midwife in their membership;
3. Random sample of midwives from the records of the midwifery organizations.

Actual sample size:
1. Competent authorities: Twelve.
2.& 3. The number of questionnaires sent to chief midwives was included in the total number sent to practising midwives from each member state.

The number of practising midwives in each state (Eurostatistiques Démographie Médicale No.180 Janvier 1991) and the number of questionnaires sent appear below, with the **Response rate:**

Member state	Midwives	Questionnaires sent	Number returned	Percentage returned
Belgium	2,382	500	352	70.40
Denmark	6,200	400	302	75.50
France	9,275	1000	113	11.30
Germany	11,000	1200	745	62.08
Greece	5,600	1000	288	28.80
Ireland	1,000	400	232	58.00
Italy	14,767	1000	274	27.40
Luxembourg	62	62	42	62.74
Netherlands	931	400	256	64.00
Portugal	1,000	1000	165	16.50
Spain	7,000	800	499	62.38
UK	31,152	1000	589	58.90
Totals		8762	3857	44.20

Interventions, outcomes and analysis:
Analysis:
Coded data analysed using SPSS.

Results:
- The data show midwifery as recognisable and definable with very strong trends in the activities of midwives across Europe even though there were differences in detail within and between countries.
- In most instances the member states of the EU entitled midwives to take up and pursue the full range of activities contained in Article 4 of Directive 80/155/EEC. However, in some this entitlement did not exist. In addition, there appeared to be a discrepancy between the practice permitted by the competent authority in some member states and the activities which were nonetheless undertaken by midwives within those countries.
- In some member states there was a lack of appropriate involvement of the midwives in the full range of activities required of midwives in Article 4 of the Directive and for which student midwives must be trained, so that although student midwives could have been exposed to the full range of activities carried out by midwives in some countries, in others they could not.
- In some countries midwives exercised appropriate levels of responsibility and independence in carrying our their role. However, in other member states there was a lack of opportunity for midwives to exercise such responsibility and independence particularly in care in labour and involvement in the conduct of normal spontaneous delivery.

Recommendations from this study:
That the following issues be addressed:
- Failure of member states to comply with the requirements of the Directive
- Discrepancy between the practice permitted by the competent authority in some member states and the activities which were undertaken by midwives
- Lack of appropriate involvement of midwives in the full range of activities required of midwives in the Directive
- Lack of opportunity in some member states for midwives to exercise an appropriate level of responsibility and independence
- The extent to which free movement of midwives whose expectation is and should be that they can fully exercise their role and responsibilities in any EU country in which they might wish to work is jeopardised in some member states.

Suggestions for further research:
- Possible replication of the study targeting a larger sample in countries where there was a low response rate (the range in this study was from 75.5 per cent in Denmark to 11.3 per cent in France)
- Further analysis of the data to provide a wider picture of the context in which midwifery practice took place, and further information on specific aspects of the activities of midwives in the different member states.
- Investigation of the changes that have taken place during the period of the project including the extent to which competent authorities might have extended the areas of practice permitted since the data were collected, the extent to which patterns of

midwifery care and the practice of midwifery might have changed in any given country during the course of the project, and social and cultural changes that might have affected women's expectations of the maternity services.

Additional relevant information:

Article 4
Directive 80/155/EEC

Member States shall ensure that midwives are at least entitled to take up and pursue the following activities:

1. To provide sound family planning information and advice;
2. To diagnose pregnancies and monitor normal pregnancies; to carry out the examinations necessary for the monitoring of the development of normal pregnancies;
3. To prescribe of advise on the examinations necessary for the earliest possible diagnosis of pregnancies at risk;
4. To provide a programme of parenthood preparation and a complete preparation for childbirth including advice on hygiene and nutrition;
5. To care for and assist the mother during labour and to monitor the conditions of the fetus in utero by the appropriate clinical and technical means;
6. To conduct spontaneous deliveries including where required an episiotomy and in urgent cases a breech delivery;
7. To recognize the warning signs of abnormality in the mother or infant which necessitate referral to a doctor and to assist the latter where appropriate; to take the necessary emergency measures in the doctor's absence, in particular the manual removal of the placenta, possibly followed by manual examination of the uterus;
8. To examine and care for the newborn infant; to take all initiatives which are necessary in case of need and to carry out where necessary immediate resuscitation;
9. To care for and monitor he progress of the mother in the postnatal period and to give all necessary advice to the mother on infant care to enable her to ensure the optimum progress of the newborn infant;
10. To carry out the treatment prescribed by a doctor;
11. To maintain all necessary records.

Publication:
European Midwives Liaison Committee (1996). *Activities, Responsibilities and Independence of Midwives in the European Union.* Report published by and available in English and in French from the European Midwives Liaison Committee (see Contact address above).

Educational studies

The study named below includes educational issues. The abstract appears on p.5 under *Clinical studies: before and during pregnancy.*

299. STUDENT MIDWIVES' EXPERIENCES OF PERINATAL DEATH

July 1992–December 1996

Sarah Davies. **Contact:** Sarah Davies, Midwifery Lecturer, University of Salford, Bury Education Centre, Talbot Grove, Bury BL9 6PH. Tel: (0161) 959 3357.

Formed part of a course. Funded by funding agency: SMA Nutrition Award, and by employer: The Northern College of Nursing, Midwifery and Health Studies, who gave 2 hours/week study leave and part of fees. 6–12 hours/week of own time spent.

Keywords: MENTORS, MIDWIFERY EDUCATION, MIDWIVES' ROLE, PERINATAL DEATH, STUDENT MIDWIVES, STUDENT MIDWIVES (ATTITUDES), STUDENT MIDWIVES (EMOTIONS)

Aims of the study:

The aim of the study is to explore the attitudes and experiences of two groups of student midwives with regard to perinatal death. One of the groups is pre-registration, the other post-registration.

Ethics committee approval gained:

No

Research design:

Descriptive, qualitative, longitudinal.

Data Collection:

Techniques used:

Interviews, questionnaires – questionnaires were about personality and death anxiety.

Time data were collected:

Three semistructured interviews during the students' course, over a period of three years.

Topics covered:

Student's attitudes to death
Experiences of death prior to midwifery training
Experiences of perinatal death and bereavement during the course
Views about midwives' role

Setting for data collection:

Mainly in the schools of midwifery.

Details about sample studied:

Planned size of sample:

Five students from each group.

Rationale for planned size:

As many as practicable. Larger sample not needed for this type of study.

Entry criteria:
Inclusion:

Two students with high death anxiety scores. Two with low scores. One with a medium score. Any other students who wished to speak about their experience.

Sample selection:

Convenience.

Actual sample size:

Five students from each group, plus other 'key informants' including qualified midwives.

Interventions, Outcomes and Analysis:
Analysis:

Content analysis, examining themes that have emerged, is ongoing.

Results:

Themes so far include:

- A marked shift from understanding the midwife's work to be concerned mainly with 'nice, normal midwifery' to seeing birth as a hazardous business both for mothers and for midwives. The use of technology, especially electronic fetal monitoring, and worries about litigation and accountability were associated with this.
- Wide variation in confidence levels of students on qualifying. Difficult mentoring relationships appeared to be a factor where confidence was low.
- A tradition of 'shielding' students from caring for bereaved families was identified and explored. Some felt that not having encountered perinatal death during training would make for problems after qualifying. This raised questions about reflective practice and the relationship between theory and practice.

Further results to follow.

Recommendations from this study:

Arrangements for mentoring need to be reviewed in order to provide improved opportunities for reflective learning. As part of the curriculum for dealing with death at birth, practising midwives could spend time discussing cases with students, 'telling stories' about situations they have been involved with.

Suggestions for further research:

The potential advantages and disadvantages of mentoring, the best use of mentoring.

Additional relevant information:

This study has now been completed, but is to be extended into a wider examination of the issues raised, at PhD level. There will be follow-up interviews of the participants, who have now qualified, and a re-examination of the data.

Publication:
Davies S. (1996) 'Divided loyalties – the problem of normality.' Editorial. *British Journal of Midwifery.* Vol. 4, No. 6, pp.285–86.

389. HIV AND MIDWIFERY PROJECT
March 1995–February 1996
David Stears, Rachel Grellier, Stephen Clift, Simon Forrest. **Contact:** David Stears, Director, Centre for Health Education and Research, Canterbury Christ Church College, Neville House, 90–91 Northgate, Canterbury, Kent CT1 1BA. Tel: (01227) 767700/782709. Fax: (01227) 780328.

Funded as integral/additional part of a job by funding agency: South Thames Regional Health Authority.

Keywords: HIV, INFECTION, INFECTION (PREVENTION), MIDWIFE TEACHERS, MIDWIFERY EDUCATION, MIDWIVES, RISK ASSESSMENT, STUDENT MIDWIVES

Aims of the study:
To assess the training needs of midwives, midwifery students and midwifery tutors with respect to human immunodeficiency virus (HIV) infection.

Ethics committee approval gained:
No

Research design:
Descriptive, qualitative, quantitative, survey.

> **Data Collection:**
> **Techniques used:**
> > Questionnaires, focus group discussions.
>
> **Time data were collected:**
> > Over a period of 12 months.
>
> **Testing of any tools used:**
> > Pilot study of questionnaires and focus group discussions.
>
> **Topics covered:**
> > Participants' knowledge levels, beliefs, attitudes and practices regarding HIV infection.
>
> **Setting for data collection:**
> > Hospitals and midwifery colleges.
>
> **Details about sample studied:**
> **Planned size of sample:**
> > Approximately 350 midwifery students, 70 midwifery tutors, and 250 qualified midwives.

Rationale for planned size:

All student midwives in training within the South Thames Region of the United Kingdom during 1995–6 and all midwifery tutors in colleges in the Region. A sample of qualified midwives in areas of the Region with high and low prevalence of HIV infection.

Entry criteria:

Inclusion:

Geographical placement within South Thames Regional Health Authority.

Sample selection:

See above.

Actual sample size:

336 midwifery students, 51 midwifery tutors and 99 qualified midwives.

Response rate:

Midwifery students 71 per cent, midwifery tutors 72 per cent, qualified midwives 36 per cent.

Interventions, Outcomes and Analysis:
Analysis:

SPSS for quantitative data from questionnaires. Content analysis of qualitative data from focus group discussions.

Results:

Although knowledge levels were generally high, less than half the students reported receiving training on HIV/AIDS. Many respondents reported disparate levels of sympathy towards HIV positive women depending on the mode of transmission. This was associated with negative images of the virus and reluctance to address issues of sexuality. Breaches of confidentiality regarding clients' HIV status were reported, and these may have resulted from fear of occupational transmission and reluctance to use universal precautions.

Recommendations from this study:

Prejudice, anxiety and embarrassment within the profession about HIV/AIDS and sexual health need to be addressed through training. The variability of provision between colleges should be reduced through development of a regional or national policy. Midwifery education, particularly in the areas of HIV/AIDS and sexual health, would benefit from the development of affective learning methodologies. Further midwifery education in these areas should be based on a 'spiral curriculum'. It has been demonstrated (Bruner, 1966) that learning is enhanced when students continually return to issues and examine them in greater depth (spiral learning), rather than studying issues on a single occasion (linear learning).

Publications:

Grellier, R., Stears, D., Clift, S., Forrest, S. (1996). *HIV/AIDS and midwifery: a study of knowledge, attitudes and practice among tutors, students and qualified midwives.* Canterbury Christ Church College: Centre for Health Education and Research. ISBN 1 899 253 20 3.

Related study:
425. ANTENATAL HIV ANTIBODY TESTING: A SURVEY OF MATERNITY UNITS IN THE UNITED KINGDOM
The abstract appears on p.17 under *Clinical studies: before and during pregnancy.*

397. STUDENT CENTRED LEARNING: TEACHERS' PERSPECTIVES

January 1993–August 1993
Sue Jacob. **Contact:** Sue Jacob, Midwifery Short Courses Coordinator, Royal College of Midwives, 15 Mansfield Street, London W1M 0BE. Tel: (0171) 872 5176 Fax: (0171) 872 5101.

Funded as part of a course by Bromley Health Authority. 2-6 hours per week of own time spent.

Keywords: ADULT LEARNERS, CONSUMER LED EDUCATION, EXPECTATIONS (STUDENT MIDWIVES'), EXPERIENTIAL LEARNING, INDIVIDUALIZED LEARNING, MIDWIFERY EDUCATION (ACCOUNTABILITY), MIDWIFERY EDUCATION (CURRICULUM), MIDWIFERY EDUCATION (MOTIVATION)

Aims of the study:
1. To explore the congruence between the institution's philosophy and that of individual teachers on student centred learning (SCL).
2. To gain an insight into teachers' interpretation and understanding of the meaning of SCL.
3. To identify the strategies, policies, teaching styles and innovations used to facilitate SCL.
4. To explore the teachers' perceived value for using SCL.
5. To highlight the restrictions of SCL.
6. To gain experience in the stages of the research process and so be able to help and encourage colleagues to undertake research.
7. To make recommendations from the findings of the study.

Ethics committee approval gained:
No. Individual teachers and the Head of the institution granted permission. It was considered beneficial for the institution to explore issues which may be raised by the study.

Research design:
Descriptive, qualitative, ethnography.

Data collection:
Techniques used:
Structured interviews and field notes of casual conversations between the researcher and teachers (permission obtained).

Time data were collected:
March–April 1993

Testing of any tools used:
> Interview schedules tested with two teachers, lecturers at the institution who were not involved in the main study.

Topics covered:
> Was SCL reflected in the educational philosophy of the institution and of the curriculum? What facilities and resources were available for SCL, including support and resources for the staff? What effect was SCL having on the workload of teachers?

Setting for data collection:
> College of Nursing and Midwifery (three of its five sites were used in the study).

Details about sample studied:
Planned size of sample:
> 12 teachers, four from each of three sites.

Rationale for planned size:
> The total number of midwifery teaching staff was small. Four from each site's team represented most areas covered in the courses.

Entry criteria:
Inclusions:
> All who were willing, available and volunteered consent.

Sample selection:
> Convenience.

Actual sample size:
> 11

Response rate:
> 11/12 = 92 per cent

Interventions, outcomes and analysis:
Analysis:
> Content analysis. Common themes and expressions were arranged into four categories:
> 1. Philosophy
> 2. Implications for the curriculum
> 2. Strategies, policies and teaching styles used to promote SCL
> 4. Physical setting for SCL.

Results:
Respondents said the philosophy of the institution and of the curriculum encouraged SCL. The institution endorsed SCL but had not resourced it or revised the structure and content of the courses accordingly; market forces were seen to be hindering SCL. The hierarchical model of management in colleges was reported not to allow the freedom of SCL. SCL gave respondents some difficulties with assessing students.

Recommendations from this study:
To create a climate for creativity and innovation and increase the confidence and competence of staff in enabling SCL, the institutions need to invest in the personal and professional development of staff.

Suggestions for further research:
A comparison of the costs of SCL with those of traditional styles of courses.

Additional relevant information:
Knowles' model of adult learning was used as the theoretical framework for SCL in the study institution.

Publications:
In preparation.

412. CLINICAL TEACHING IN MIDWIFERY: AN EXPLORATION OF MEANINGS
August 1992–March 1993
Christine Bewley. **Contact:** Mrs. Chris Bewley, Senior Lecturer, Middlesex University, Faculty of Health Studies, 10 Highgate Hill, London N19 5ND. Tel: (0171) 288 5932. Fax: (0171) 288 5103.

Formed part of a B.Ed (Hons) course in education. Course funded by employer and by the King's Fund. 2–6 hours/week of own time spent.

Keywords: CLINICAL TEACHING, EXPERIENCE (STUDENT MIDWIVES'), MIDWIFE TEACHERS (EXPERIENCES), MIDWIFERY EDUCATION, STUDENT MIDWIVES (ATTITUDES), STUDENT MIDWIVES (EMOTIONS), SUPPORT (PROFESSIONAL)

Aims of the study:
To determine what is meant and understood by the term clinical teaching, to explore student midwives' experiences of clinical teaching, and to ascertain whether the transition from student to midwife influences approaches and attitudes to clinical teaching.

Ethics committee approval gained:
No. Not required at the time.

Research design:
Descriptive, qualitative, phenomenology.

> **Data collection:**
> > **Techniques used:**
> > > Tapes of semistructured interviews, field notes and the researcher's reflective diary.
> >
> > **Testing of any tools used:**
> > > Each participant's interview was discussed with her in conjunction with a transcript of the interview and, with all but one of the participants, a copy of the study findings.

Topics covered:
>   See study aims.

Setting for data collection:
>   A College of Health Care Studies attached to a large maternity unit.

Details about sample studied:
Planned size of sample:
>   Eight

Rationale for planned size:
>   Manageable by one researcher in the time available.

Entry criteria:
Inclusions:
>   Student midwives and midwives qualified within the previous year who consented to participate.

Sample selection:
>   Convenience

Actual sample size:
>   Eight; four student midwives and four midwives.

Response rate:
>   N/A

Interventions, outcomes and analysis:
Analysis:
>   Used techniques described by Hycner (1985) and Burnard (1991) specifically modified for phenomenological research.

Results:
The main findings of the research suggest that clinical teaching was understood to be a didactic, teacher led activity which occurred in the clinical area but away from mothers and babies. Students experienced other significant learning in the clinical area that arose almost by accident as they went about their work. This learning was viewed negatively, and not always capitalised upon. The transition from student to qualified midwife, although exciting, was stressful; informants felt unsupported in their role, and considered themselves ill-prepared for the task of mentorship. Midwife teachers were valued in the clinical area, but they were considered to be out of touch and in a hierarchy of work, theirs was considered the least important.

Recommendations from this study:
The findings lend support to two models of teaching which would enable the midwife teacher to legitimate her teaching activities in the clinical area, and place education and service on a equal footing. These are the lecturer/practitioner and the personal tutor.

Bewley, C. (1995) 'Clinical teaching in midwifery: an exploration of meanings'. *Nurse Education Today*, 15, pp.129–35.

417. EVALUATION OF ASSESSMENT STRATEGIES IN THREE YEAR PRE-REGISTRATION MIDWIFERY PROGRAMMES

January 1995–December 1998

Diane M. Fraser. **Contact:** Diane M. Fraser, Head of Division of Midwifery, School of Nursing and Midwifery, University of Nottingham, A Floor, Queen's Medical Centre, Nottingham NG7 2UH. Tel: (0115) 970 9279. Fax: (0115) 970 0878. Email: Diane.Fraser@nottingham.ac.uk.

Funded by employer as part of a job and part of a course. 2–6 hours/week of own time spent.

Keywords: EXPECTATIONS (WOMEN'S), EXPERIENCE (PARENTS'), EXPERIENCE (WOMEN'S), MIDWIFERY EDUCATION (CURRICULUM), MIDWIFERY EDUCATION (DIRECT ENTRY), MIDWIFERY EDUCATION (EVALUATION), MIDWIFERY EDUCATION (RECRUITMENT), STUDENT MIDWIVES (ATTITUDES)

Aims of the study:

Evaluation of the effectiveness of three year pre-registration midwifery programmes in terms of outcome to inform curriculum development.

Exploration of the notion of competence to try to establish the goals for student midwives to achieve and when and how achievement of them is determined.

Ethics committee approval gained:

Yes

Research design:

Descriptive, qualitative and quantitative, action research.

Data collection:

Techniques used:

Documentary analysis, student profiles in particular.

Interviews with students, midwife assessors and midwife teachers in 1995 complete cohort. Observation of student class evaluations.

Written evaluations.

Questionnaires to 1996 completers.

Interviews with women, antenatally and postnatally.

Case note review.

Time data were collected:

1995 and 1996 completers in the month prior to completion.

Case notes prior to interviews.

Women: at first hospital visit, during postnatal stay, and during third week postpartum.

Testing of any tools used:
>Interview schedules based on earlier work.
>Questionnaires piloted with 5 students elsewhere.

Topics covered:
>Student midwives:
>>Preparation for role/course effectiveness
>>Value of assessments/assessment scheme generally
>>Validity and reliability/role of teachers and assessors
>>Achievement of UKCC Rule 33/Activities of Midwife.
>>Areas for improvement.
>>Strengths/weaknesses
>>Confidence, competence, qualities, potential aspirations.
>Mothers:
>>Most important attributes of a competent midwife
>>Most important factors in recruitment and selection of student midwives.

Setting for data collection:
>Hospital, University, women's homes.

Details about sample studied:
Planned size of sample:
>All 22 students who completed training in 1995, all 1996 completers.
>40 women.

Rationale for planned size:
>Students' experience is very varied, being gained on seven sites, therefore all included.
>Advised by supervisor that 40 women would be a feasible and adequate number for the study.

Entry criteria:
Exclusions:
>Women under 16 years old, living outside the area, or with a pregnancy not likely to be viable judging from GP s letter.

Sample selection:
>All students completing training in 1995 and 1996.
>Convenience sample of women.

Actual sample size:
>22 students from 1995 cohort. 1996 not yet known.
>41 women invited to take part.

Response rate:
>21 students from 1995 cohort. 40 women.

Interventions, outcomes and analysis:
    Analysis:
        In progress. Manual, pre-specified plus emerging themes.

Results:
In preparation.

418. AN OUTCOME EVALUATION OF THE EFFECTIVENESS OF PRE-REGISTRATION MIDWIFERY PROGRAMMES OF EDUCATION
October 1993–October 1996

Diane M. Fraser, Head of Division of Midwifery; Roger J. L. Murphy, Dean of Faculty of Education; Michelle Worth-Butler, Research Midwife. **Contact:** Diane M. Fraser, Head of Division of Midwifery, School of Nursing and Midwifery, University of Nottingham, A Floor, Queen's Medical Centre, Nottingham NG7 2UH. Tel: (0115) 970 9279. Fax: (0115) 970 0878. Email: Diane.Fraser@nottingham.ac.uk.

Commissioned by The English National Board for Nursing, Midwifery and Health Visiting (ENB). 2–6 additional hours/week of own time spent.

Keywords: COMPETENCE, EXPERIENCE (MIDWIVES'), EXPERIENCE (PARENTS'), EXPERIENCE (STUDENT MIDWIVES'), MIDWIFE TEACHERS (EXPERIENCES), MIDWIFERY EDUCATION, MIDWIFERY EDUCATION (EVALUATION), MIDWIFERY EDUCATION (PRE-REGISTRATION)

Aims of the study:
The overall aim of this two stage project was to evaluate programme effectiveness. A case study approach, supplemented by other methods, enabled the researchers to develop a model of competence in midwifery and to identify factors which facilitated or inhibited effective assessment.

Stage 1 aimed to evaluate the immediate effectiveness of the three year pre-registration midwifery programme of education, including:
- examination of the philosophy, theoretical framework, design and content of curricula;
- identification and development of new tools for the assessment of outcomes;
- assessment of the intended and actual outcomes in terms of knowledge, attitudes, competencies and skills.

Stage 2 aimed to evaluate the effectiveness of these programmes in the light of one year's practice, including:
- effectiveness one year on in terms of knowledge, attitudes, competencies and skills;
- identification of continuing educational needs;
- retention rates, career patterns and career intentions of midwives qualified via three year route.

Ethics committee approval gained:
No. Ethical guidelines were provided for institutions who then decided whether to participate.

Research design:
Descriptive, qualitative and quantitative, survey, case study.

Data collection:
Techniques used:
Document analysis, interviews, observations, questionnaires, diaries, focus groups, literature review, discussion group summaries.

Time data were collected:
Throughout the project.

Testing of any tools used:
Questionnaires and interview schedules tested and re-tested, questionnaires with ten people and interview schedules with 2–3 for each group.

Topics covered:
Students and midwives: assessment, competence, confidence, evaluation, effectiveness of programme, gaps/further education needs.
Women: perceptions of midwifery care.

Setting for data collection:
Education settings, hospitals, women's homes.

Details about sample studied:
Planned size of sample:
Six geographically spread case study institutions (out of 23 institutions offering pre-registration programmes and willing to participate).

Rationale for planned size:
Largest feasible sample.

Entry criteria:
Inclusions:
Commenced three year pre-registration midwifery programme between august 1991 and April 1992.

Exclusions:
Self-exclusion

Sample selection:
According to pre-determined criteria to represent a good cross section.

Actual sample size:

Six sites. 39 students from the six case study sites have formed part of a longitudinal study.

Response rate:

N/A

Interventions, outcomes and analysis:
Analysis:

Emerging themes. Main themes coded and re-analysed to identify specific issues within each of the original themes. A double blind approach was adopted to test reliability of categories. Computer software: Text-Base Alpha.

Results:

Results are in preparation and publication of the main report is expected in March 1997.

Recommendations from this study:

Recommendations will be to the ENB to assist with policy making.

Mountford, B., Fraser, D.M., Murphy, R. J. L. (1995). 'An interpretative comment on twenty three pre-registration curricula documents. A summary paper prepared as part of an ENB commissioned report'. The EME Project: University of Nottingham.

Worth-Butler, M., Murphy R. J. L., Fraser D. M. (1994). 'Towards an integrated model of competence in midwifery'. *Midwifery* 10(4): pp.225–31.

Worth-Butler, M., Murphy R. J. L., Fraser D. M. (1995). 'Recognizing competence in midwifery'. *British Journal of Midwifery* 3(5): pp.259–62.

Fraser D. M., Murphy R. J. L., Worth-Butler, M. (In press). 'A model of competence: the consumer's perspective'. *British Journal of Midwifery.*

Management studies

All these studies have a bearing on clinical issues. Among those listed as *Clinical studies* many include management issues, especially those named below:

407. Self-medication: another step in maternity wards discarding their traditional ethos of illness and patienthood (abstract p.51)

419. Home birth (abstract p.74)

305. BALMORE PARK MOTHERS AND MIDWIVES SCHEME, PARTNERS IN CARE, PILOT PROJECT
April 1994–April 1996

Caroline Simpson, Sharon Kearns, Ruth Moynes, Annette Weavers, Linda Ayres, Jackie Harrington. **Contact:** Caroline Simpson, Senior Midwife (Community), Sandleford Hospital, Newtown Road, Newbury, Berkshire RG14 7ED. Tel: (01635) 32500 Ext. 3317. Fax: (01635) 41463.

Funded as integral/additional part of a job. 2–6 hours/week of own time spent.

Keywords: AUDIT, CARE COMPARISONS, CONTINUITY OF CARE, CONTINUITY OF CARER, EXPERIENCE (WOMEN'S), MIDWIFERY STAFFING (STRUCTURES), TEAM MIDWIFERY

Aims of the study:
To establish if caseload midwifery, applied to a partnership of three (2.8 whole time equivalent (WTE)) midwives attached to a specific GP practice, is a feasible and successful way of achieving the Changing Childbirth objective that '75 per cent of all women should be cared for in labour by someone they have come to know in their pregnancy'.

Ethics committee approval gained:
Yes

Research design:
Experimental, qualitative, quantitative, survey.

Data Collection:
Techniques used:
Questionnaire to mothers; retrospective and prospective audits of outcomes; midwives' reflective diaries.

Time data were collected:
Questionnaire: up to one year after delivery.
Audit: retrospective for women in the GP practice who delivered in 1993 and prospective for women who delivered during the project (1994–95).
Reflective diaries: throughout the project.

Topics covered:
Questionnaire to mothers: continuity of care, venue of care, satisfaction.
Audit: age and parity, length of labour and analgesia used, complications and interventions, mode of delivery, Apgar scores, feeding methods, admission to neonatal unit.

Reflective diaries: Kept so that the project midwives could aggregate and feed back their experiences of working on the project. Topic areas decided by themselves and included job satisfaction, on call arrangements, work and family/social life, working relationships, self-management.

Setting for data collection:
Community

Details about sample studied:
Planned size of sample:
Approximately 120 women per annum. The three project midwives.

Rationale for planned size:
Number of women from the GP practice who deliver annually.

Entry criteria:
Inclusion:
All women receiving maternity care in the practice.

Exclusion:
Women from the practice who deliver in other units.

Sample selection:
All mothers from the practice who gave birth between April 1993 and March 1995.

Actual sample size:
119 sets of casenotes for the retrospective audit.
159 mothers who gave birth during 1994–95.

Response rate:
All the casenotes. 60 per cent of the women. All three midwives.

Interventions, Outcomes and Analysis:
Interventions used:
Women have direct access to a named midwife or her partner and the choice of home assessment in early labour, labour care by a known midwife, and early home discharge (2 hours). Women can be accompanied for induction of labour or planned caesarean section.

Main outcomes measured:
Women's satisfaction, clinical outcomes and midwives' reflections.

Analysis:
Content analysis for user's satisfaction questionnaire. Audit entered onto Microsoft Access database, which can be queried according to item measured. Midwives' reflections summarised by themselves.

Results:

The prospective audit of all the project women showed that over 80 per cent received care in labour from one of the three project midwives.

The results of the users survey indicated that from their perspective, all the objectives of the project were met. Women who received care from the partnership of three midwives during the project reported:

- greater satisfaction with antenatal care
- better communication between midwife and mother
- greater confidence about birth matters
- feeling more relaxed during labour
- feeling more in control of events, through knowing their carer and establishing a relationship of trust
- feeling more personally supported

in comparison with a sample of women throughout Berkshire who received conventional care during the same period (Birch, K., Poole, W. (1996): see Additional relevant information).

Home assessment in early labour was associated with reduced length of time in hospital and less analgesia in labour. Further results on clinical outcomes and on midwives' reflections are in preparation.

Recommendations from this study:

Address information deficit perceived in Berkshire overall, and to a lesser degree in Balmore Park.

Additional relevant information:

A comparative survey of a randomized sample of 450 women receiving conventional care in West Berkshire has been undertaken and published. These women received the same postal questionnaire as in the Balmore Park survey. A response rate of 69 per cent was achieved.

Birch, K., Poole, W. (1996). 'Mothers and Midwives: Prospects for Changing Childbirth' University of Keele, Centre for Health Planning and Management. ISBN 1-900580-03-9.

377. EVALUATION OF MIDWIFERY TEAMS IN WEST ESSEX
November 1994–September 1995

Corinne Camilleri-Ferrante, Chris Todd, Morag Farquhar. **Contact:** Morag Farquhar, Research Associate, Health Services Research Group, Institute of Public Health, University of Cambridge, Forvie Site, Robinson Way, Cambridge, CB2 2SR. Tel: (01233) 217744/330329. Fax: (01223) 330330. eMail address: mcf22@medschl.cam.ac.uk.

Funded as integral/additional part of a job by commissioning agent: Department of Obstetrics and Gynaecology, Princess Alexandra Hospital, Harlow, Essex.

Keywords: CONTINUITY OF CARE, GENERAL PRACTITIONERS, HEALTH VISITORS, JOB SATISFACTION, MIDWIVES, OUTCOMES, TEAM MIDWIFERY, WOMEN'S VIEWS

Aims of the study:
1. To describe West Essex's community midwifery teams.
2. To assess the satisfaction levels of those working in and with the teams.
3. To describe the experiences and satisfaction levels of women from West Essex using the teams.
4. To describe the clinical outcomes of births to women cared for by the teams.
5. To establish the number of midwife contacts women using the teams have both antenatally and intrapartum.

Ethics committee approval gained:
Yes

Research design:
Descriptive, qualitative, quantitative, survey, case control study.

Data Collection:
Techniques used:
Postal questionnaires to service users (or interviews with women who had a stillbirth, a baby with abnormalities, a baby on special care baby unit, or who had a postnatal stay >10 days).
Postal questionnaires to staff, interviews with key professionals.
Clinical data collection by midwives.
Audit sheet of women's antenatal and intrapartum contacts with midwives.

Time data were collected:
Minimum of ten days postnatally.

Testing of any tools used:
Questionnaires, interviews and clinical data form were piloted during December 1994.

Topics covered:
Service users:
- antenatal care
- intrapartum care
- postnatal care
- demographics

Midwives, GPs and health visitors:
- job satisfaction
- views of team midwives
- demographics
- previous posts
- qualifications

Setting for data collection:
Hospital, client's home, urban, rural.

Details about sample studied:
Planned size of sample:
Minimum 1200 women: all who used the team midwifery service 1/1/95–30/06/95 plus three control groups.

Rationale for planned size:
Size adequate for analysis.

Entry criteria:
Inclusion:
Six month census sample of those who used the team midwifery service.
Control group 1. Women delivering at study unit but cared for antenatally and postnatally by teams from the other unit.
Control group 2. Women delivering at other unit but cared for antenatally and postnatally by community midwives from neighbouring unit.
Control group 3. Women delivering at other unit but cared for antenatally and postnatally by one of the midwife teams.

Exclusion:
Women who had no antenatal care.
Out of area women, other than control group 1.
Women whose babies were to be adopted.

Sample selection:
Census

Actual sample size:
1335/1520 women.

Response rate:
Women: 88 per cent to user survey, 95 per cent for clinical data and 85 per cent for audit.
Staff: 95 per cent community midwives, 84 per cent hospital midwives, 78 per cent GPs and 83 per cent health visitors.

Interventions, Outcomes and Analysis:
Main outcomes measured:
Clinical outcomes
Satisfaction of service users and staff.

Analysis:
Mann Whitney U test, Chi-square test, Kruskal-Wallis test, Fisher's Exact test, using SPSS for windows.

Results:

For the purposes of this abstract, one point for each of the study's aims has been selected from the many results reported.

1. Midwives, General Practitioners, Health Visitors and users of the service all said the size of the West Essex teams and caseloads should be reviewed.

2. 45 per cent of community midwives felt the scheme was working well in West Essex compared with 19 per cent of hospital midwives. Over half the study group GPs and 70 per cent of the health visitors said they would go back to working in the way they did before the introduction of team midwifery, most commonly because communication and liaison had been better.

3. The control group of women who received the most traditional care (usually seeing one or two midwives, in conjunction with their GPs, for their antenatal and postnatal care and being delivered by a probably unknown midwife) were the most satisfied with their antenatal care. There were no differences between the samples with regard to their reported satisfaction with care during labour and delivery, postnatal care in hospital of postnatal care at home.

4. Process and outcome data included a higher than expected percentage of women having team care classified as high risk (29 per cent). There were no differences between the samples in terms of whether the same midwife remained with them throughout labour and delivery.

5. Inconsistencies were found between midwives' and users' recordings of whether a woman had been delivered by a midwife she had met before.

Selected recommendations from this study:

1. Reconsider the number of midwives on the teams and their caseload, to overcome the apparent detrimental effect of the size of the teams on the antenatal and postnatal continuity of midwifery care in West Essex.

2. Steps to ameliorate interprofessional liaison are suggested.

3. Note the views of women regarding the quality of relationships they reported developing with their midwives.

4. Steps to improve consistency of evidence based advice and care are suggested.

5. Consider offering women a choice between team care and care based on one or two midwives. The former offers the possibility of a known midwife at delivery, whilst the latter is more likely to result in one or two midwives offering ante and postnatal care, but little possibility of a known midwife at delivery.

Suggestions for further research:

Further research is needed to identify women's priorities with regard to the possible choice outlined above, between team care and care based on one or two midwives. Any steps which are taken to bring about improvements in care must be evaluated and monitored to assess their effectiveness.

Additional relevant information:

The report of this study has been launched and papers for publication are in preparation (August, 1996).

Farquhar, M., Camilleri-Ferrante, C., Todd, J. (1995). 'Continuity of care in maternity services: women's views of one team midwifery scheme'. British Sociological Association's Medical Sociology Group Conference, University of York, 22–24 September 1995

Farquhar, M. Camilleri-Ferrante, C., Todd, J. (1996). 'Keeping your perspective: women's views of one team midwifery scheme'. Changing Childbirth-the first two years: Conference, Kensington Conference Centre, London, 19 June 1996.

384. GETTING CONSUMERS' VIEWS OF MATERNITY SERVICES
January 1991–July 1992
Sue Wardle. **Contact:** S. A. Wardle, Epidemiologist, Department of Public Health and Health Policy, South Staffordshire Health Authority, Mellor House, Corporation Street, Stafford, ST16 3SR. Tel: (01785) 52233, Ext. 5165. Fax: (01785) 50684.

Funded as integral/additional part of a job by employer: Mid Staffordshire Health Authority, and by Milupa Baby Foods.

Keywords: ANTENATAL CARE, BREASTFEEDING, CHOICE, CONSUMER SATISFACTION, LABOUR (CARE), MATERNITY SERVICES, POSTNATAL CARE

Aims of the study:
To assess satisfaction with maternity services in one health authority.

Ethics committee approval gained:
Yes

Research design:
Descriptive, quantitative, survey.

> **Data Collection:**
> > **Techniques used:**
> > > Postal questionnaire.
>
> > **Time data were collected:**
> > > 7–8 weeks after delivery.
>
> > **Testing of any tools used:**
> > > Used established tool, OPCS survey package.
>
> > **Topics covered:**
> > > Antenatal care
> > > Antenatal classes
> > > Information
> > > Care during labour and delivery
> > > Postnatal care in hospital and community

Setting for data collection:
Client's home.

Details about sample studied:
Planned size of sample:
All women in the area who delivered during an 8 week period in April and May 1991. Names forwarded from Child Health Computer System.

Rationale for planned size:
Planned to receive sample of 400. Assumed 75 per cent response rate and 2 per cent ineligible and estimated that there would be 533 births in 8 weeks. In fact there were 596 births in the chosen 8 weeks.

Entry criteria:
Inclusion:
All mothers resident in the health authority who delivered during the study period.

Sample selection:
Some oversampling took place to achieve larger samples from some hospitals.

Actual sample size:
639 questionnaires sent.

Response rate:
513 returned, 80.3 per cent.

Interventions, Outcomes and Analysis:
Analysis:
SPSSPC statistical computer package.

Results:
Approximately three quarters of women were satisfied with the care they had received from the maternity services, but several areas were highlighted for improvement. The main criticisms were lack of information, attitude of some staff, and staff having too little time to talk. Fewer women than expected were breast feeding, both in hospital and at home. None reported having problems with which they wanted more help than they received.

Wardle S. Getting consumers' views of maternity services. (1994) *Professional Care of Mother and Child* 4(6) Aug/Sept pp.170–74.

Related study:
424. A MODIFIED REPLICATION OF THE OPCS SURVEY OF WOMEN'S EXPERIENCE OF CHILDBIRTH USING A POSTNATAL QUESTIONNAIRE
The abstract appears on p.80 under *Clinical studies: women's views.*

385. CHANGING CHILDBIRTH: IMPACT ON STAFF AND SERVICE USERS
February 1995–June 1997

Soo Downe, Sheila McFarlane. **Contact:** Soo Downe, Research Midwife, Maternity and Gynaecology Research and Audit Office, 3rd Floor, Derby City Hospital NHS Trust, Uttoxeter Road, Derby, DE22 3NE. Tel: (01332) 340131 Ext 5070. Fax: (01332) 290662. Email:derbymatgynae@dial.pipex.com

Funded as integral/additional part of a job by funding agencies: Department of Health (Changing Childbirth funds) and Southern Derbyshire Health Commission. Also by employer: Derby City General Hospital NHS Trust. 2–6 hours/week of own time spent.

Keywords: CARE COMPARISONS, CHANGING CHILDBIRTH, CHANGE (ORGANIZATIONAL), CHOICE, COMMUNITY MIDWIVES, CONSUMER OPINION, CONTINUITY OF CARE, COST EFFECTIVENESS, GENERAL PRACTITIONERS

Aims of the study:
Phase one:
1.1. To establish the effect of the change process on the staff (midwives, GPs, consultant obstetricians and managers) involved in Changing Childbirth teams (pilot teams).
1.2. To establish whether multiple parameters of maternal experience/satisfaction differ between cases and controls.
1.3. To establish whether clinical outcomes differ between cases and controls.
1.4. To establish whether financial outcomes differ between cases and controls.
Phase two:
2.1. To identify and address staff training needs as perceived by the staff themselves and by the service users.

Ethics committee approval gained:
Yes

Research design:
Qualitative, quantitative, survey, case control study, action research.

Data Collection:
Techniques used:
1.1. Interviews, diaries, two psychometric scales, questionnaires.
1.2., 1.3., 1.4. Questionnaires, routine clinical data.
2.1. Focus groups, questionnaires, interviews.

Time data were collected:
Various times depending on aspect being addressed.

Testing of any tools used:
Staff questionnaires: face validity by research team, pre-pilot and pilot prior to distribution.

Psychometric scales were pre-tested: (Glasgow Midwifery Process Questionnaire (1995) Midwifery Development Unit, Glasgow Royal Maternity Hospital; Warr, P. (1990) Measurement of wellbeing. Occupational Psychology vol 63 pp 193-210).

Women's questionnaires: based on OPCS and MacArthur et al (MacArthur, C., Lewis, M., Knox, E.G. (1991) Health after Childbirth. University of Birmingham, HMSO), tested and amended over the last four years.

Interview schedule: face validity by research team, consistency maintained by using only one interviewer.

Setting for data collection:

Hospital, health centre, GP surgery, client's home, staff homes.

Details about sample studied:
Planned size of sample:

1.1. At least one GP from each pilot and control practice (n=15). All pilot (n=17) and control (n=11) midwives. Labour ward (n=8) midwives, randomly selected from all labour ward midwives. Three consultant obstetricians, randomly selected from all eight consultant obstetricians.

1.2., 1.3., 1.4. All women cared for by pilot teams (approximately 500), each matched to two controls on five potentially confounding variables (approximately 1000).

2.1. 15 x 8 women for focus groups.

Rationale for planned size:

1.1 Maximum coverage without jeopardising opportunities for staff to share experiences.

1.2., 1.3., 1.4. All women booking with the scheme in the first 14 months. Two matched controls for each woman on the basis that the response rate may be lower from controls.

2.1. Fifteen groups identified by women and staff as being important. No more than eight participants per group to allow for effective group dynamics.

Entry criteria:
Inclusion:

1.1. All pilot and control midwives. Representative GPs as agreed by each GP practice.

1.2., 1.3., 1.4. All women cared for by pilot teams, and matched controls.

2.1. Focus groups: depending on criteria for each group.

Exclusion:

Unwillingness to participate. Women who suffered pregnancy loss or loss of the baby for any reason (miscarriage, termination, perinatal death, SIDS, adoption or fostering). Maternal death.

Sample selection:

    1.1.   Interviews, diaries and psychometric scales: all pilot and control team midwives, and a random selection of labour ward midwives. Interviews only: one GP from each pilot and control practice, and a random selection of consultant obstetricians.

    1.2., 1.3., 1.4. Total pilot population matched to two controls on five variables. Each case woman is matched with the next two women booking in the same month, in alphabetical order, who match all five criteria.

    2.1.   Purposive sampling of eligible postnatal women delivering at the study unit within one year prior to the focus group.

Actual sample size:

Not yet fully known.

Interventions, Outcomes and Analysis:

Interventions used:

Pilot teams: With the aim that 75 per cent of women shall have a known carer in labour, a team midwife accompanies each woman into hospital for any attendance on labour ward, regardless of risk. This is currently being modified so that non-labouring women might not be accompanied, e.g. for an overnight prostin. Prior to the project 9 per cent of women in the study unit had a known carer in labour.

Main outcomes measured:

Phase one:

    1.1.   Change demonstrated in views of staff over a longitudinal assessment of diary entries, three interviews and the psychometric scales.

    1.2.   Comparison of degree of fulfilment of expectations between pilot and control groups and a range of experiential outcomes.

    1.3.   Percentage of women in pilot and control groups having a known carer in labour, and a range of clinical outcomes.

    1.4.   The relative cost of the care given to the cases and controls (type of economic analysis to be determined after outcomes are known).

Phase two:

    2.1.   Self-assessed levels of competence and confidence in identified areas before and after staff training.

Analysis:

    1.1.   Team mean scores for psychometric tests. Content analysis of diaries and interviews.

    1.2., 1.3. Descriptive and inferential statistics.

    1.4.   Economic analysis (Cost Benefit Analysis, Cost Minimisation Analysis, Cost Utility Analysis) with sensitivity analysis.

    2.1.   Content analysis and descriptive statistics.

Results:
Results from the initial interviews pointed to pilot teams' concerns about training needs and excessive on-call. Both issues are being addressed organizationally.

Interim analysis of the Glasgow Midwivery Process Questionnaire demonstrates that the pilot team with an initially high score has reduced this markedly over time, and the other team, initially scoring low, has now markedly improved. Reasons for this change will be explored in the final report.

Phase one of the project has been extended to March 1997, and results will be available by June 1997. At the interim point, 64 per cent of pilot women met a known midwife in labour.

Phase two is not now due to complete until June 1997. Focus groups with women are complete, and reveal that staff attitudes and hospital based postnatal care are key areas for staff development.

404. EVALUATION OF A NEW COMMUNITY-LED MATERNITY SERVICE
November 1993–April 1996

Debra Kroll, Senior Midwife; Anne Fleissig, Research Fellow, Department of Epidemiology and Public Health, University College London Medical School; Mark McCarthy, Director of Public Health, Camden and Islington. **Contact:** Debra Kroll, Senior Midwife, Research and Development and Outpatient Services, Obstetric Hospital, University College London Hospitals, Huntley Street, London WC1E 6AU. Tel: (0171) 380 9719 Fax: (0171) 380 9565.

Funded as integral part of a job by a Locally Organized Research Scheme of North East Thames Regional Health Authority. Up to 2 hours/week of own time spent.

Keywords: COMMUNICATION, COMMUNITY MIDWIVES, CONTINUITY OF CARE, CONTINUITY OF CARER, MATERNITY CARE EXPERIENCE, MIDWIVES' ROLE, PERCEPTIONS OF TEAM MIDWIFERY, STAFF ATTITUDES

Aims of the study:
To evaluate the implementation, effectiveness and acceptability of a community-led integrated maternity service. Community-led care is defined as appropriate care by community midwives and general practitioners during pregnancy, birth and the puerperium, with routine hospital care kept to a minimum.

Ethics committee approval gained:
Yes

Research design:
Descriptive, qualitative and quantitative, survey, case series.

Data collection:
Techniques used:
Case note review; questionnaires to recent mothers, community midwives, general practitioners (GPs), consultant obstetricians and labour ward midwives; routine data from off-duty rota forms. Women who did not speak and write in English had the written questionnaires and their answers translated by interpreters who went to their homes.

Time data were collected:
Case note review: retrospective
Survey of recent mothers: six weeks postnatally
Survey of staff: approximately 18 months after implementation of the new service.

Testing of any tools used:
Case note review: care planning forms specifically designed for the study.
Maternal questionnaire piloted with 20 women.
GP questionnaire finalised after consulting with GPs working outside the local area.

Topics covered:
- Case note review: Plan of care compared with actual care and reasons for changes. Continuity of carer, referrals and outcomes, and place of care.
- Survey of mothers: experiences of antenatal, intrapartum and postnatal care and views about choice and continuity of care.
- Survey of community midwives: Organisation of services; questions about the care of women, continuity and communication with other professionals, views on the structure of teams, workload, support and job satisfaction.
- Survey of GPs: Choices given to women, antenatal care arrangements, communication with other professionals, impact of community-led maternity care on GPs and women.
- Survey of consultant obstetricians: Views about community-led care and arrangements, number of visits to hospital antenatal clinic, referrals and communication.
- Survey of labour ward midwives (core staff): Views about continuity of care, role of community midwives, communication.

Setting for data collection:
Case notes from an urban hospital. Postal surveys.

Details about sample studied:
Planned size of sample:
500 sets of case notes. Surveys: 250 mothers, 28 community midwives, 60 GPs, 6 consultants, 8 labour ward core staff midwives.

Rationale for planned size:

Case notes of all mothers meeting the study criteria. Surveys: half the mothers, all community midwives allocated to provide their care, all GPs in the study's local area, all consultant obstetricians in the study unit, and all core labour ward midwives.

Entry criteria:

Inclusions:

Women resident in South Camden who booked at the study unit for maternity care between 1.10.93 and 31.3.94.

Exclusions:

Case notes of women who moved out of South Camden in early pregnancy or cancelled bookings. Postal survey excluded women who moved out of South Camden postnatally and those whose baby had died. GPs not involved in antenatal care and those who had been working locally for less than six months were excluded.

Sample selection:

Convenience. Postal survey: systematic 1:2 sample of eligible mothers (alternate women were selected from lists sorted by booking date).

Actual sample size:

453 women, 524 initially recruited and 71 excluded by study criteria. 28 community midwives, 60 GPs, 6 consultants, 8 labour ward midwives.

Response rate:

Postal survey of women:	146/195	= 75 per cent
Community midwives:	25/28	= 89 per cent
GPs:	49/60	= 82 per cent
Consultants:	6/6	= 100 per cent
Labour ward midwives:	6/8	= 75 per cent

Interventions, outcomes and analysis:
Analysis:

Data analysed using SPSS. Statistical tests include Z test for difference between proportions, T test for difference between means, Chi square test for trends.

Results:

Eighty-five per cent of women planned to have community-led care including 8 per cent who had initial complications. Only 3 per cent transferred to full hospital care during pregnancy. Women having community-led care saw an average of three community midwives antenatally. 68 per cent had some intrapartum care from their 'named' team of community midwives, and 31 per cent were looked after by their team throughout labour and delivery. 53 per cent of women surveyed had met at least one of their intrapartum midwives prior to labour. 22 per cent had postnatal home visits from five or more midwives. The full complement of community midwives was not achieved for 17 per cent of on call shifts. In summary, the proportion of local women who were able to have antenatal and intrapartum care from community midwives increased under the new service, but the expected continuity of carer was not achieved. Many community midwives were disappointed, but most women were highly satisfied with their care, even when they did not receive the continuity of carer anticipated. The main concern identified by other professionals was insufficient communication.

Recommendations from this study:

- Community led maternity care as described was a satisfying option for the majority of women both with and without complications.
- Women who develop complications antenatally may not need to transfer to full hospital care if community midwives have access to specialist opinion and facilities where necessary.
- Although the majority of women had access to local antenatal care from staff they got to know, the named community midwives and teams found it difficult to provide comprehensive care, particularly to the women who developed complications, and so priorities need to be established.

Suggestions for further research:

Further research is required to compare alternative models of care and to examine their costs and cost effectiveness.

Additional relevant information:

Many more results and recommendations are available in the full report.

Fleissig, A., Kroll, D. (1996). Evaluation of community-led maternity care in South Camden, London. London: Health Services Research Group, University College London Medical School (internal report).

Sources of funding for new MIRIAD studies

The sources and amounts of funding for studies varied considerably. Sources of funding are listed if they contributed at all to a study; they may not have supported the whole study. Many studies received no formal funding and researchers themselves provided the resources for others, both in time and money.

Sources of funding for studies numbered 394 onwards are listed here in alphabetical order. The studies to which they have contributed are listed below their name.

Anglia and Oxford Regional Health Authority
Infant weaning: lay and professional accounts of the weaning process

Baby Lifeline
Evaluation of maternal physiologic response to mechanical milk expression following preterm delivery

Bromley Health Authority
Student centred learning: teachers' perspectives

The Edwina Mountbatten Trust
Activities, responsibilities and independence of midwives within the European Union

The English National Board for Nursing, Midwifery and Health Visiting
An outcome evaluation of the effectiveness of pre-registration midwifery programmes of education

The European Union, Small Grants
Activities, responsibilities and independence of midwives within the European Union

Evian/Birthright
A study exploring midwives' education in, knowledge of and attitudes to nutrition in pregnancy

Health Education Authority
Systematic review of research evidence of effectiveness of current interventions aiming to promote healthier eating in women of childbearing age, and those who are pregnant

Health Promotion Research Trust, Cambridge
Exploring differences in women's experiences of pregnancy and early motherhood

The Hospital Savings Association Charitable Trust
Differences in perineal trauma between Bengali and Caucasian women
Women's experience of waterbirth

Institute for Social Studies in Medical Care
Obstetricians' views on prenatal screening and diagnosis

King's Fund
Midwives without children: a phenomenological study of relationships
Clinical teaching in midwifery: an exploration of meanings

Mid Trent College of Nursing and Midwifery
Evaluation of assessment strategies in three year pre-registration midwifery programmes

NHS Executive (Mother and Child Health)
Detection of fetal abnormality at different gestations: impact on parents and service implications

North East Thames Regional Health Authority
Evaluation of a new community-led maternity service

Pinderfields NHS Trust
A modified replication of the OPCS survey of women's experience of childbirth using a postnatal questionnaire

Royal College of Nursing, Midwifery Society
Antenatal HIV antibody testing: a survey of maternity units in the United Kingdom

Royal College of Obstetricians and Gynaecologists National Birthday Trust Fund
Home birth

The Royal London Hospital
Some beliefs about colostrum and reasons for its omission to the newborn among women from Bangladesh

The Royal National Pension Fund for Nurses
Activities, responsibilities and independence of midwives within the European Union

Scottish Office (Chief Scientist's Office)
Handling of premature neonates: study using time-lapse video

The Smith and Nephew Foundation
Women's experience of waterbirth

Author index

Name	Study no.	Page no.

Name	Study no.	Page no.
Ralph, Ann	426	3
Rankin, Jean	381	19
Renfrew, Mary J.	283, 370	32,41
Richmond, Helen	400	72
Rogers, Jane	235	45
Rowett, Valcrie	424	80
Ruby, Christine	425	17
Sames, Lesley	370	41
Scanlen, Siobhan	370	41
Simpson, Caroline	305	111
Siney, Catherine	425	17
Sleep, Jennifer	370	41
Smith, Angela	420	91
Smith, Lynn	399	78
Solomou, Wendy	430	15
Spencer, S.A.	403	63
Spiby, Helen	416	5
Stanisstreet, Martin	374	2
Statham, Helen	430	15
Stears, David	389	99
Swain, Ian	350	30
Swayne, Pippa	350	30
Symon, Andrew	413	66
Telfer, Florence M	356	7
Todd, Chris	377	113
Truesdale, Ann	199, 235	47,45
Van Asten, Hedwig	370	41
van Teijlingen, Edwin	426	3
Wardle, Sue	384	117
Watson, D.	368	9
Weavers, Annette	305	111
Wilcox, Mark A.	356	7
Wilson, Brenda J.	426	3
Winter, Cathy	370	41
Wood, Juliet	235	45
Worth-Butler, Michelle	418	107
Wraight, Ann	419	74
Yerby, Margaret	396	36

Keyword index

THE MIDWIFERY RESEARCH DATABASE: MIRIAD

To claim your **free** six-month subscription to the **new** MIRIAD Register please complete and return this card.

Title: _____

Name: _____

Address: _____

_____

_____

_____ Post code: _____

Tel: _____

Do not
affix
stamp

Books for Midwives Press
Freepost WA1836
Hale
Cheshire
WA15 9BR